JOURNEY TOWARD WHOLENESS

A SPIRITUAL ENCOUNTER WITH PROSTATE CANCER

R. CARROLL STEGALL

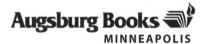
Augsburg Books
MINNEAPOLIS

To Clarice, whose love renews me daily

To Cyndi, who helped me make sense out of chaos

JOURNEY TOWARD WHOLENESS
A Spiritual Encounter with Prostate Cancer

Copyright © 2004 R. Carroll Stegall. All rights reserved. Except for brief quotations in critical articles or reviews, no part of this book may be reproduced in any manner without prior written permission from the publisher. Write to: Permissions, Augsburg Fortress, Box 1209, Minneapolis, MN 55440.

Large-quantity purchases or custom editions of this book are available at a discount from the publisher. For more information, contact the sales department at Augsburg Fortress, Publishers, 1-800-328-4648, or write to: Sales Director, Augsburg Fortress, Publishers, P.O. Box 1209, Minneapolis, MN 55440-1209.

Scripture passages are from the New Revised Standard Version of the Bible, copyright © 1946, 1952, 1971, 1989 by the Division of Christian Education of the National Council of the Churches of Christ in the USA. Used by permission.

ISBN 0-8066-4595-4

Cover design by David Meyer
Book design by Michelle L. N. Cook
Cover art from Getty Images

The paper used in this publication meets the minimum requirements of American National Standard for Information Sciences—Permanence of Paper for Printed Library Materials, ANSI Z329.48-1984. ♾ ™

Manufactured in the U.S.A.

08   07   06   05   04   1   2   3   4   5   6   7   8   9   10

CONTENTS

FOREWORD

BY CYNDI ALTE

For some time, beginning in October 1994, those of us who worked with Clarice Stegall had been keeping close track of her husband, Carroll. From the first test results showing an elevated PSA (an indicator of prostate cancer), Carroll was in our prayers. For the months before his final diagnosis of prostate cancer, through his surgery, and into his recovery, a host of persons surrounded him with prayer support. It was not just our relationship with our churches and our God but our concern for Carroll that created such intense support and care.

Carroll's personal management of his cancer fascinated all of us. He brought an almost perfect integration of physical, spiritual, and mental care to his way of dealing with his diagnosis and subsequent treatment regime. Carroll studied his medical condition with the same attention to detail that his personal physician used. He considered carefully how his relationship with God might affect his physical state. He was deliberate in his observation of his personal thought processes.

From my perspective of having been a registered nurse for ten years and an ordained minister for ten years, it would have been easy to think of him as a perfect case study in holistic medicine. But our relationship has been anything but a case study.

When Carroll first called to ask if I would consider spending some time with him talking about his cancer and the new path his faith was taking because of it, I did not hesitate. From the beginning Carroll was honest, open, and completely frank. In an almost innocent, childlike way, he wanted to know what was happening to his spirit and to his mind as his body was changing. So his question to me, "Will you guide me through this?" evoked my immediate, "Yes!"

My role as guide changed as Carroll's needs changed. I was a cheerleader: *You can make it through this tough moment . . . hour . . . day . . . week . . . month. Just get beyond your feelings. We will handle the rest.* I was a challenger: *That dream means more than what you are thinking. Be brave enough to face what it is telling you.* I was a doubter: *You cannot be going through all of this and not feel angry. There is not one human being on earth who would not be mad as hell at what is happening to them.* I was a mother: *It really will be okay. Maybe not this instant, but I will try to make it better for you.* I was a pastor: *God is in the midst of this with you. After all, God watched God's son die, never leaving his side. God will not leave you.*

Two significant events in our "counseling" (I hesitate to use the word, as this was not counseling in its traditional sense. It was much more.) shaped our relationship. Early on, when Carroll was struggling with fear, I sensed that he needed reassurance that I would always be there for him. That feeling came from my understanding that pastors often represent God to those with whom we relate. Mindful that I am *not* God in any sense, I do have the blessed assurance of knowing someone is there for me. I gave Carroll my beeper number. Although it may seem like a minor offering, my beeper number is available only to my family, the church secretary, and one friend.

Carroll took me up on the offer to be available to him at any time, calling at times when he needed to hear another human voice assuring him that he could make it through the day.

Telling Carroll that he would be part of a fairly small number of people privy to my attention did just what I had hoped it would. Within a short time, Carroll was able to transfer the assurance that he could call on me anytime to the knowledge that God was available to him at any time. It was a privilege to be a part of that kind of "God work"—the kind that convinces people that God is at work all the time for all people.

The second shaping event in our time together was Carroll's request that I be part of a team that would pray for him. I had already been praying for him, but his question this time was specific. Would I pray that his PSA (at that time an exceptionally high 67.0) would decrease four points a day until the next time he was tested? Although I had never been part of such a particular prayer request, I was eager to support him by honoring his wish.

For some years I have been in the habit of passing the names of people I love and for whom I have concern to God before I take a bite of any meal. So at breakfast, noontime, and dinner—and every other time that I eat during the day—Carroll's name and specific request were whispered to God along with the names of my family and friends.

Frankly, at times I doubted the PSA levels would decrease through the power of the "four-point prayer," as I came to call it. Fortunately, my doubt was not the mitigating factor in Carroll's PSA level. As it decreased in such a dramatic, inexplicable manner, I came to realize that this was a miracle beyond my medical knowledge. What happened this time that is so different from other cases? My spiritual insight tries to clarify it and cannot. Prayers are offered daily for those who are sick or dying, but no miracle occurs for them. Is Carroll any different from others who are prayed for? Once again I face the realization that there are things in the world we will never understand and for which we will find no explanation. And once again I am grateful that I am not charged to have all knowledge or all wisdom.

Carroll's persistence in connecting his physical battle with his spiritual journey was heartening, enlightening, inspiring, and challenging. He continues on his admirable path of integrating his body, mind, and spirit in a holistic manner, trying to become what God would want him to be. Being a part of his journey has been a privilege that few ministers have in their careers. I am grateful to have been a part of Carroll's illness and, more important, grateful to have been a part of his search for wellness.

PREFACE

BY CLARICE STEGALL

What do you say when the person you love more than anyone else in the world finds out he has cancer—prostate cancer? What do you say when the best treatment option is surgery, which most likely will render him impotent? How do you deal with the shock, the hurt—for him even more than for yourself? How do you handle the distress of further treatment—radiation, then hormone therapy—the latter of which takes away even his interest in sex? How do you cope with his feeling ill, being unable to cope, and being greatly depressed without letting yourself fall apart? Where do you get the strength to let him lean on you when you are not sure you can remain standing yourself? What can you do to let him know that in spite of all these things, you still love him completely, as he is, and that you always will? How can you help him believe that you believe in him and in his love for you, even if there must now be different ways of expressing that love? How can you join him in praying for complete recovery, without also praying "God's will be done"? And how can you pray for God's will, knowing the results might not be what you want? How do you even express your thoughts about any of this?

One's future is always uncertain, no matter how carefully one plans. But facing mortality—one's own or that of one's beloved—makes the future seem even more uncertain. I don't even want to think about what might lie ahead for Carroll, for us; but in reality I know I must. Many things need to be dealt with: housing, income, health care, all sorts of practical things—plus the most important issue of living each day to the fullest.

I have never doubted Carroll's love for me, nor mine for him. The full physical expression of our love waited for our wedding night, at which time we began to learn how to fulfill and be fulfilled in the deepest intimacy. We have continued to learn through all of our marriage. And now we are learning new ways of fulfillment. We have learned that the depths of love do not require sexual expression, as special as that can be, for love to be valid, full, and complete. Just being together becomes more precious; special times become more special.

Carroll's writing of this chronicle has been cathartic. His openness and honesty on two radio programs about how he is dealing with his experience with cancer has been a strengthening experience. I have seen him become very much at peace as he has accepted God's healing in ways not before experienced.

So, how am *I* handling all this? What do I *feel?* Fear. Frustration. Sadness. Loss. Uncertainty. *How* do I feel? I don't know. I started this response by asking a lot of questions. I don't have all the answers. I pray daily for strength and courage to deal with this life-changing challenge—and the other family and job concerns with which I also must deal. I do the best I can. And I try to remember that someone said, "It's not over 'til it's over." I keep reminding myself that God won't give us more than we can bear. But as Mother Teresa said, "Sometimes I wish he didn't trust me so much."

ACKNOWLEDGMENTS

Many thanks to those who read the manuscript and offered valuable suggestions, including Rev. Dr. George W. Campbell, a cancer survivor and longtime friend; storyteller and cancer patient Nancy de Vries (now deceased); Janice Lawless; Philip Snodgrass, MD; Joel R. Stegall, PhD; Judith Turner; Helen Zebarth.

Thanks also to members of the medical community who provided assistance in correcting and verifying the accuracy of the medical information: Matthew Davis, MD; James Ehlich, MD; Arve Gillette, MD; James Kluzinski, MD; Keith Logie, MD; Richard Rhodes, MD; Bruce Roth, MD; David Scheidler, MD.

Multitudes of friends from around the country have shown support with calls, letters, cards, and prayers.

Rev. Cynthia (Cyndi) Dell Alte deserves special mention as the person who put me in touch with the holistic nature of healing.

How can I just say "thank you" to my beloved Clarice? Her role as proofreader for this manuscript was invaluable. But that was a minor event. To her and to Jon, Joi, and Jeremy, whose lives have been altered by my illness, who have given me reason to live fully every day, I love you.

INTRODUCTION

Why write yet another first-person prostate cancer account? Of the many writings on prostate cancer that have sprung up in the past few years, few take in the way spirit, mind, body, and relationships intertwine. Those forces exert powerful roles in disease and in wholeness. I have set out to explore, with the reader, that intertwining. We will discover that the question of wholeness goes far beyond the specifics of a particular disease. My prostate cancer is your breast cancer is his death is her despair.

In the process we will talk about dreams. Because stress can play a role in the development of cancer, we will talk about events that may at first seem removed from the cancer experience. We will talk about relationships with other people. We will talk about a relationship with God.

To accomplish those tasks, I must make clear the particular lens through which I see. I am a Christian who believes that all people are children of God. Though much of my training is academic, I believe that wisdom comes through inspiration, or intuition, channeled through the subconscious. I am by profession a musician and storyteller, with no claim to medical authority. I have checked out medical information with doctors who deal with the subject and with recognized reference works. To protect confidentiality, I have in several cases disguised names.

I am a private person. I do not easily share sexual and anatomical intimacies. But because the disease affects the functions of reproduction and elimination, the story must include specific descriptions of those functions.

Joy and humor may spring from serious situations without trivializing the situation. When I lose my sense of humor, I'm dead! So I choose to live.

CHAPTER 1

BEGINNINGS

C ancer doesn't hear prayer." My friend's words stopped me in mid-sentence. He is a physician who has seen plenty of cancer. He is a spiritual person. He is an intellectual whom I highly respect. "People pray and pray, and their cancer keeps growing. Others never pray, and the cancer goes away."

"Then, why pray?"

"Pray for strength to endure. But no matter how much you pray, cancer has a mind of its own."

I was particularly vulnerable to his remarks right then. For the past year, I had run the gauntlet of prostate surgery, radiation, and hormone therapy. I had read everything I could get my hands on. I had talked with anyone who would not run away from me. I had tried to follow doctor's orders. Many people were praying for me. Yet signs of cancer just would not go away. "Cancer doesn't hear prayer?" Neither my friend nor I could know at the time that those four words would propel me into the adventure of exploring for myself mind-body-spirit relationships.

My first direct encounter with prostate cancer had come two years earlier, when a colleague had undergone a radical prostatectomy. Soon after he returned to work, he had asked me, "Have you had your PSA tested?"

"My what?"

"PSA. It's a new blood test that indicates prostate cancer. Every man over fifty ought to have it done every year."

When I had my next physical, I asked my family physician, Dr. Jack Lukowski, if he was checking the PSA. He said he was, but because the readings had been favorable, had not mentioned them.

"What is it?" I wanted to know.

"Prostate Specific Antigen." It is an enzyme that is produced only by the prostate. A normal reading is 4.0 (in nanograms per milliliter [ng/ml]) or below. If it is high, it can mean that the prostate is enlarged, is infected, or is cancerous. I remembered that my colleague's reading had been around 14 before his surgery. Also that when he came back to work, he wore a catheter bag on his leg. I would not have been aware of it except that he had a habit of squeezing the bag to see how full it was.

It would be some time before I would know much more. But I eventually found out that PSA, produced by the prostate gland, is also produced by prostate cancer. Recent research has discovered traces of PSA secreted by other organs.[1] Thought for years to have no measurable effect on its own, it now is seen to contribute to several functions, including turning semen from a viscous state to liquid after ejaculation.[2] So the PSA is not the problem. Too much PSA indicates an abnormal function. Further tests are required to determine the nature of the abnormality.

A few days after the physical, we got a call from Dr. Lukowski's office. My PSA was 14.7. He made an appointment for me to see Dr. Donald Shiller, a urologist, for a biopsy. Dr. Shiller is a brisk young man with a voice like a laser. He has a way of pausing after making an important statement, nodding his head and staring at you. At first I thought his eyes would pop out of his head. He told me exactly what he would do. I did not much like what I heard: "Using an ultrasound probe as a guide, we will run a needle up your rectum, puncture through the intestinal wall into the prostate gland, and dig out tissue samples. We will get samples from six different areas of the prostate. But we will give you a hefty dose of Valium, so you should be too relaxed to care. You will hardly remember the procedure later." Then he paused, nodded his head, and gave me that bug-eyed stare. He was wrong on all counts. He performed the biopsy on November 30. I don't remember conversations in the lobby on the way out. However, I made an intimate acquaintance with each of the six probes. I thought a bee had flown up my rectum.

A week later we got the report: all six samples were negative. Clarice said: "Is that good? I can never remember which way it goes."

"Yes, it's good. That means they found no cancer. But he wants me back for a recheck in six months. An elevated PSA usually means something is wrong, although there are sometimes false readings."

Christmas came. Clarice and I are both church musicians. Since 1987 we had been working in two separate churches, so we always had two sets of Christmas music to prepare. Our youngest child, Jeremy, had for several years been wrapped up in seasonal concerts with the Indianapolis Children's Choir. Our daughter, Joi, always had a long agenda of personal and family holiday goals. And when Jon, our eldest, was home, he filled the house with the aroma of his gourmet cooking.

We set our family holiday concert record the year that the five of us were in fourteen performances, all on different music, in twelve days. But this year was different. Clarice had resigned her church music position in June, and was doing only substitute organ playing. For the first time in nearly twenty years, she did not have a church music year to plan. Advent is her favorite season, but with no Advent music to plan, she approached Christmas with dread.

Jeremy, now sixteen, had aged out of the Indianapolis Children's Choir that spring, so he was not involved in any Christmas concerts. Joi could not come home because she was in college at Oklahoma State University and was working full-time. Jon had come up from Charlotte, North Carolina, at Thanksgiving time, so he was unable to get back for Christmas. The main event of this Christmas was when a car hit our beagle, crushing her right rear foot. Veterinary bills cost the price of a fancy Christmas.

In February 1995 Clarice began a long-term position as interim organist at Saint Andrew Church, on the west side of Indianapolis. By mid-April Saint Andrew offered us permanent positions, Clarice as organist and handbell director, I as music director. We could now work together the way we used to. This change meant leaving two major support groups. For eight years I had been music director at the historic Downey Avenue Church, in the Irvington section of Indianapolis. During that same time, I had directed the Indianapolis Maennerchor. Founded in 1854, it is the oldest men's chorus in the country. I had nurtured them musically, and they had nurtured my faith.

Nature thwarted the plan to personally present letters of resignation at the board meetings of the two organizations, both of which fell on Monday evening, May 1. Late that afternoon, probably due to stress, stomach flu blew my insides apart. Instead of saying good-bye to my friends in person, I crawled into bed. Little did I realize how soon and how much I was going to need the fellowship that was now discontinuing.

The stomach flu kept me at less than half speed (except on my dashes to the bathroom) for about two weeks. Just as I was getting over the flu, it was time to start a round of antibiotics to prepare for the next PSA test. Dr. Shiller wanted to make sure there was no infection to throw the blood test askew. The antibiotic made me sick all over again.

Being sick for a whole month awakened a sleeping dragon.

CHAPTER 2

IMMUNE SYSTEM AT WAR

What was your life like two years before you were diagnosed?" When I read that question in a survey of cancer patients, my mind reeled backward. The first hints of chronic illness had knocked on my door long before I even knew anyone with prostate cancer. Cancer can sneak in when the immune system fails to do its job or becomes overwhelmed. It can infiltrate our bodies when we are under great stress.

In the spring of 1992, three years before my cancer diagnosis, I had contracted what felt like a low-grade flu. It had produced a lot of coughing, dizziness, and fatigue, though no fever. In June I gave a singing-and-storytelling performance for a music camp at Broad Ripple High School in Indianapolis, where I taught voice in the Center for Performing and Visual Arts. By the end of the performance, I became winded and nearly passed out.

It was time to see the doctor. Dr. Jack Lukowski is a no-nonsense physician who believes in going at treatments aggressively. The symptoms sounded like pneumonia, so he prescribed Biaxin, which he called the "atom bomb" for pneumonia. While on the medication, I continued my summer private voice-teaching schedule.

In July Clarice and I went to the annual Association of Disciple Musicians (ADM) church music workshop. Because we attend this workshop every summer, we have developed lasting and deep friendships among the regular participants. This year, teaching a class on the spiritual nature of storytelling kept me going. However, dizziness and coughing increased. When we got back, the doctor ordered another round of Biaxin.

In August, Jeremy, just shy of turning fifteen, went with me on an eight-day car trip around my home state of North Carolina. We visited relatives and long-time friends, saw places where I had lived as a child, and took in places that were famous for history, folklore, and ghost lore. I even sang on Sunday at the church I had attended in high school. Though it rained every day, it was, for me, a dream trip. It also allowed for some much-needed closeness with my youngest child.

But I never felt normal. I fatigued easily and coughed a lot. Something needed to be done. I did not want to make a big issue out of it, because I was able to keep working and do all the things I had to do. But being a singer and not being able to take a deep breath without coughing or running out of air on short musical phrases were sure signs of trouble. I had prided myself on being able to sustain a long musical phrase, even after blowing out much of my air. I had used it as a trick to impress my students occasionally. By now, however, I had quit singing except when demonstrating for my students.

So it was back to Dr. Lukowski when we returned to Indianapolis. Jack told me: "I'm putting you on my worry list. It is time to get you bronked."

"Bronked? What does that mean?"

"Bronchoscopy. They'll put a fiber-optic lens down your windpipe to see what is causing this congestion. Something is in there that acts like pneumonia but does not respond like pneumonia. I'm setting you up with Dr. Rick Holmes, a pulmonologist. He'll take care of it."

Pulmonologist. Lung specialist. The only thing I knew about specialists was that it usually took weeks to get appointments and that they charged by the minute. Next thing I knew, however, I was sitting in Dr. Rick Holmes's office, looking around the waiting room at people on oxygen and otherwise appearing to be very sick. Dr. Holmes was fortyish, short, trim, with a winning smile and an anachronistic flattop haircut. He put my X rays up on the viewing screen and pointed out scattered spots that indicated "infiltrates" of unknown nature in the lungs. "We will run a tiny tube through your nose and down your windpipe. The tube will have a light, a camera lens, and a probe with which we can take samples of tissue. You will be conscious enough that you can assist us, but you will not remember a thing when the procedure is over."

This proved to be the first of several times I would have to clean out my digestive system. The doctor didn't want me throwing up on him while he was looking down into my lungs. What would he find? Asthma? Tuberculosis? Cancer? I was too numb to ask. I had felt run down so much of the time for the past four months that I actually looked forward to being knocked out, so I could get a few good hours of sleep.

Bryon Rose, my pastor from Downey Avenue Church, was on hand, along with Clarice, when the nurse started the IV. One minute we were chatting. The next minute I was opening my eyes in recovery. A nurse asked if I felt I could get up. I said, "I could, but I don't want to." And promptly went back to sleep for another hour.

On the next visit to Dr. Holmes, he reported no evidence of asthma, TB, or cancer. What he did find was an infiltrate that indicated "interstitial lung disease," inflammation of the lining of the lungs. The inflammation generated pus. The pus is what I was coughing up. Though Dr. Holmes could describe the condition, he could not diagnose it. He then referred me to a rheumatologist.

"What's the connection? Rheumatism? I don't even know what that is."

He explained that a rheumatologist deals with connective tissue diseases such as arthritis and lupus. He had taken a batch of blood tests that did not show positive for any of the usual connective tissue diseases, so he needed a connective tissue specialist to find out what the culprit was. When he mentioned *arthritis,* I remembered that I had felt arthritislike pain in my right wrist and forearm, but had not connected it with the "lung crud."

More blood tests. This time the lab technician took fourteen vials of blood samples. I figured he had some under-the-table deal with Dracula. Meanwhile, Dr. Holmes set me up with Dr. Joshua Henson, his rheumatologist of choice. By now Clarice was going to all the appointments to take notes. We were getting too much new information too fast to absorb it, much less process it. I certainly needed her—and her shorthand skills—when we met Dr. Henson, a smooth-skinned, pompadour-haired, precise young doctor, who spoke with the clarity and personal touch of a computer. He scanned my chart and pointed out that the only disease I had tested positive for was Sjögren's syndrome. He then asked me about symptoms such as extreme dryness of the mouth and eyes, inflamed gum tissue, and so on. Nothing matched. "You don't show any symptoms related to Sjögren's, but you test positive for it. You test negative for lupus, but you show symptoms of internal lupus, such as fatigue and lung inflammation."

"What do we do?"

"Let's try Plaquenil. It was developed early in this century as a treatment for malaria, but it has also proven helpful with arthritis, lupus, and related diseases. Nobody knows how it works. We only know that it does. It fell out of use for a number of years because, being a quinine product, it tasted awful. But now they have developed a coating that makes it tasteless. Just don't bite into one!"

"But when someone asks me what I have, what do I tell them?"

"Tell them we don't know. But it doesn't really matter what you call it; the treatment is the same."

He went on to explain that results would not show up for a week or so, but that the fatigue, dizziness, and coughing should become less frequent. "Don't stop when you start feeling good. With the medication you can expect to lead a pretty normal life. Without it you will become debilitated."

It was a momentous occasion the Thursday night in October 1992 when I took the first two 200 mg tablets of Plaquenil. Once started, it was for the duration. The next time I saw Dr. Holmes and reported Dr. Henson's findings, he exclaimed, "Plaquenil? I haven't heard of that since medical school!" He did suggest a name for the condition, however. He said, "Who knows? Someday it may be called 'Stegall's Syndrome'!"

Joi was a freshman in college. She sent home leaflets about lupus. The materials kept talking about "autoimmunity." I asked Dr. Holmes if that meant that the immune system has failed, like it does with leukemia and AIDS.

"No, it means the immune system turns on itself. It's like the castle guard that is supposed to protect the castle. The guards turn and start fighting one another, letting the bad guys walk right in. That's why you may be more susceptible to flu, et cetera, than other people."

Autoimmunity can strike anywhere. In this case it chose the lungs as the place to camp out. The constant battle of my own cells against my own body was creating the inflammation. The struggle of mind with body also generated depression. Plaquenil did help, but the chronic cough and periodic fatigue continued for most of a year. One of my Maennerchor friends, John Schild, revealed that he had taken Plaquenil for years to treat his arthritis. He then offered to hold a healing service for me, saying that he no longer had to take pain medication for his arthritis since he had been anointed with oil for healing. I appreciated his sincerity, but declined. Anointing with oil sounded to me too much like the tent-meeting healing services the Holy Rollers used to hold across the highway from our house in eastern North Carolina.

Coughing, dizziness, depression, and fatigue continued until the summer of 1993. That year our national church music workshop was to be held in July at Stetson University, in DeLand, Florida. Our twenty-fifth wedding anniversary was coming up in August, so our children paid for a Bahamas vacation. Because neither of us had ever been to the Caribbean, Clarice and I were thrilled with the prospect and overcome by the children's generosity. We planned to take the Bahamas trip immediately after the workshop.

Meanwhile, family crises claimed our attention far more than did my physical problems. We were soon sucked into a series of events that threatened our family stability, safety, and friendships. Details of this adventure are another story for another time. I mention it here to indicate the extreme stress we all endured. If it did not set up at least one of us for becoming sick, it missed a golden opportunity.

Still reeling from those events, Clarice and I prepared to leave for our long-awaited Florida-Bahamas vacation. As we collected our various stashes of money for the trip, we discovered that a sizable stash of money was missing from our lockbox. Jeremy, Joi, and Jon all offered to give us money to cover the loss. We searched and asked many questions, but found no hint of the missing cash. It was gone, without a trace, forever.

By the time we packed for Florida and the Bahamas, we dreaded what might happen while we were gone. Now we needed minds and spirits mended even more than bodies. At the workshop one of our daily worship experiences was to be a healing service. The idea planted by John Schild months earlier finally became a determination to give it a try. In the weeks leading up to the workshop, I prepared to present myself for healing. Having never done anything like this, I was both eager and apprehensive. Was I just succumbing to wishful thinking, or, worse, the hocus-pocus of the tent revivals I had known about since I was a child? I even hesitated to tell Clarice. But the need was too great; I had to try.

We arrived in DeLand, Florida, to enthusiastic reunions with friends we had made over the years of annual participation in this workshop. Yet I dared not talk with anyone about the planned healing service. In spite of my reservations, at the prescribed time, I presented myself to the ministers for laying on of hands and anointing with oil. I asked for healing from my mysterious illness and a resolution of the conflicts surrounding our family.

My good friend and pastor from a former church, Warren, and another pastor who came to be a warm friend, June, performed the ceremony for me.

My skepticism about spiritual healing urged me to keep track of the results. I had no coughing, fatigue, dizziness, or depression from that day on. I said nothing to anyone, not even Clarice, until I had gone for six months without any symptoms. But I still stayed on the medication.

The family turmoil would take more time to resolve. I will come back to it later.

CHAPTER 3

DIAGNOSIS CANCER

I continued with no ill effects for two years. We now return to the spring of 1995, when the stomach flu weakened my system and the prebiopsy antibiotic threw it off balance. Then all those earlier symptoms returned. Often, always while I was alone, I would stumble around feeling dizzy, unable to focus my attention, gasping for breath, breaking into panicked sobs, and occasionally screaming out for help into the empty house. There was rarely any external motivation, except allowing myself to be rushed. I would cough every time I lay down and every time I got up from bed. It was much like it was before I had started the Plaquenil in 1992. Only now it was worse.

Such was my basic physical and emotional state when Dr. Shiller took the second PSA on May 30, 1995. On Friday, June 2, came the report: the PSA level had risen to 37.1, double what my colleague's had been before his surgery. Dr. Shiller fixed me with that bullfrog stare and announced that we had to do another biopsy. I said, "Okay, Donald, but be sure you give me more dope this time." He scheduled it for June 7. Clarice went into the room with me. He doubled the Valium, confident this dosage would knock me out. No such luck. All six stabs drilled into my permanent memory. A further annoyance: I had to abstain from sex for several days after the biopsy because of blood in my urine, stools, and semen.

On Tuesday, June 13, I called Dr. Shiller to get the biopsy results. I figured it would be negative like the last time. Not so. All three samples from the right side were positive, indicating a malignancy that rated a 5 on an activity scale (Gleason scale) of 1 to 10. That meant the cancer was moderately aggressive. Further tests would determine whether it was contained within the prostate. The next step was to check in at the hospital the next day for a bone scan. The doctor wanted to make sure there were no "hot spots," indicating cancer in the bones. Then I was to report back to him on Thursday.

I immediately called Clarice. "How do you feel?" she wanted to know. "Like crawling in a hole somewhere?"

"No, I feel like the other shoe just dropped. We have been hanging on a 6/4 chord[3] too long. We've finally come to a cadence." All morning, even before the call, I had been singing in my brain Jean Berger's musical setting of "I to the hills lift up mine eyes; from whence shall come mine aid?" based on Psalm 121. When a major crisis hits, I usually get an overwhelming desire to sleep. But not this time. I took a long walk. The second part of the psalm started working on me: "My help comes from God, who made heaven and earth." I had known Berger's composition since college. Only after it had aged for thirty years in the cellar of my mind and thrust itself back into consciousness did I realize that the composer had used all twelve tones of the chromatic musical scale in this tune. He had excluded no note of the musical alphabet. The words of the psalm reached me on one level. The music now touched another. If I am going to write my new song, I can leave out no note of my life's alphabet. The new song must include all of my knowledge, all of my reason, all of my experience. That same psalm was to rescue me again after surgery.

Having lived with chronic disease for three years, checking in the next day for the bone scan was just routine. "Oh, you want to take another test? You want me to jump through hoops? Okay."

The upcoming visit to Dr. Shiller, however, generated major jitters. He had already outlined the basic options for prostate cancer: surgery, radiation, hormone therapy. Up to now it had all been academic. Those things only happened to other people. But that phone call on Tuesday had dragged us across an invisible threshold. There was no going back. Clarice got off work early to go with me to the next appointment on Thursday, June 15. We had to wait for most of an hour before the doctor could see us. I had worked up a good fester of impatience by the time he finally showed up. He apologized, saying that he had been dealing with another patient in a similar circumstance to mine, and he needed to give each patient all the time they needed. I knew then that we were in for a rocky road.

He reviewed the choices. Surgery and radiation had comparable results,[4] but if we chose radiation and it did not take, he could not go back to do surgery because the prostate would be "cooked" and surrounding tissue would also be damaged. They could insert radioactive pellets directly into the gland (brachytherapy). This procedure had shown some success, but it was too new to judge long-term results. He did not do the brachytherapy.

Freezing the cancer with liquid nitrogen (cryosurgery) would be another possibility.[5] The drawback: it is hard to confine the effects. They could zap more than what is intended.[6]

Hormone therapy is not considered a first-line treatment. It is used as a follow-up, but is not effective in getting at the fundamental growth. I did not ask how hormone therapy worked. I would find that out in due time.[7]

Dr. Shiller described the surgery. He would make an incision from my navel to the pubic bone.

I interrupted, "Can you avoid cutting through the *rectus abdominis?* I am a singer. That abdominal muscle is where I get my major singing support."

"We don't cut the muscle itself. We cut the tendons that bind the muscles together, then spread them apart."

That sounded okay so far. Then came the tough part.

He reminded us that the prostate, about the size and shape of a walnut, is attached to the large intestine and wraps around the urethra. "We will cut away the entire prostate gland and the seminal vesicles. If possible we will save at least one of the bundles of sex nerves that trigger erection.[8] Not all patients are candidates for nerve sparing. If there is evidence, or suspicion, of cancerous cells under the nerves, they cannot be spared safely."

By now I was drowning. Couldn't he just core out the prostate and get the bad cells, like the lumpectomies they do for breast cancer? Then I realized. *Foolish boy,* I said to myself. *Most prostates are much smaller than most breasts. The lumps they excise from a breast may be larger than your whole prostate!* This little internal debate continued while Dr. Shiller went on with his explanation.

"If we can spare one set of nerves, you may still be able to have an erection, and an orgasm of sorts, but there will be no fluid to ejaculate." I would have to wear a catheter for several weeks, and could have continued incontinence. Radiation may be needed as a follow-up.

Clarice asked about chemotherapy. He answered, "Chemotherapy has not shown itself to be very effective with prostate cancer."

Dr. Shiller urged us to get a second opinion. He gave us the name of a local urology practice that did the radioactive implants.

When we left the doctor's office, we took a long walk along Fall Creek Parkway. At first I could not talk at all. Lost forever would be one of Garrison Keillor's Four Great Joys of Life: Learning, Sweet Corn, Sex, and Walking Rightly with Your God.[9] Finally I managed to croak out: "I know you love me, and nothing will make me stop loving you. But not to be able to show you . . . ," then burst out in spasms of crying.

Her answer was as gentle as a spring breeze. "You show me in so many ways, in everything you do. This must be, for a man, as scary as breast cancer is for a woman."

On Friday I called other urology practices. They did not have time for something as trivial as a second opinion. One receptionist said that unless I was a regular patient of that practice, I would have to wait six weeks for an appointment. Another would not disclose over the phone whether their practice actually performed the implant procedure. I finally said, "To hell with it," and went with my gut feeling, that Donald Shiller could do as good a job as anyone. That gut feeling would be confirmed again and again in the coming months.

We have had more bodywork done on our cars than I would like to admit. Every car we have driven has, at some time, found its way to the sick bay at MAACO. As a consequence I have become well acquainted with the owners, a Lebanese family. Mohammed and Jay Sayah are co-owners. They immigrated in the mid-1980s. They and their wives all have MBAs. They looked for the best franchise deal they could find. After careful shopping, they bought into MAACO, a national bodywork franchise. Their wives, children, nephews, and nieces all work there.

Shortly after my cancer diagnosis, I took one of our cars to their body shop after a minivan had smashed into the driver-side door while Clarice was driving. Jay Sayah invited me back to his office while he calculated the cost of repair. On the wall was a plaque inscribed in Arabic. I asked him to translate it.

He replied, "It's hard to say in English, but I'll try." He wasn't satisfied with his off-the-cuff translation. When I returned several days later to pick up the car, he handed me a sheet of paper with the Arabic inscription, a syllabic transliteration, and an English translation. Here is what it said:

Hatha min fadio rubbi This is from the bounty of God
Allah jella jellaloh Allah, glory and praise be to him.

He attached a note with the translation: "*llah* means 'god.' For example, Jesus said, 'llahi llahi lima sabachtani' ('My god, my god, why have you forsaken me?'). *Al llah* means 'the god.' It is read in Arabic as *Allah*, and became a proper name for the creator." Jay, his wife, and Mohammed all knew of my upcoming surgery.

He explained further that the inscription encompasses an affirmation that everything that happens is according to the will of Allah. "This I do not believe. This I know."

I was skeptical of his statement. It sounded too fatalistic to one who passionately believes in free will. But I had no doubt of his certainty—a certainty I had never experienced in my own faith. I later asked Jay, "Where does free will come in?"

"Free will? Free will means that you choose how you react." He was warming up. "Free will means that you do everything in your power. Free will means that you struggle and fight." He stood, paced around his office. "Free will means that, when you have done everything you can possibly do . . ." He stopped, turned, and looked me in the eye, "then you say to God, 'All right. I've done everything I can do. The rest is up to you.'"

❋

Now it was time to take my friend up on his offer for an anointing service. If it had worked for my lung crud, perhaps it would work for cancer. Saturday morning, June 17, I met with four of my friends, plus Pastor Paul of Cross and Crown Lutheran Church. Pastor Paul's words and actions were reassuring. By reminding us that God's healing may not be our healing, he removed the anxiety of "your faith wasn't strong enough" if the cancer is not removed. I still felt self-conscious about verbalizing my expectations, but Pastor Paul gave me no choice.

So I swallowed hard and prayed, hoping I was not lying: "I believe God will heal me. I believe that, if God chooses, the cancer will be gone when the doctor goes in. But it is always God's will, not mine."

Saying the prayer out loud did something. It transformed my thinking. The ceremony does not pretend to work magic. Instead, it is a means for focused prayer. Five men then laid their hands on my head. As they prayed I felt power surging through my body.

Coming out of the spiritual high of that morning, I arrived home with my emotions sticking out six feet in all directions and began making phone calls. The next day was to be my first Sunday directing the choir at Saint Andrew Church, and the first time in twenty years that I would direct a church choir with Clarice as organist. We had worked together in many contexts. I had sung in her choirs. She had conducted me as soloist in her performances. She had accompanied community choruses that I had founded in two communities. She had accompanied my solo performing. She had been vocal director of musicals I had conducted and performed in. She, many times, had accompanied and helped coach my private voice students.

Now we had been working separately, directing choirs in different churches for eight years. On this Saturday morning, as I sat in the kitchen making phone calls regarding the Saint Andrew choir, Clarice kept calling out from the sewing room with questions I was supposed to ask. I had already asked them, but she had not heard. After the third or fourth interruption, I finally yelled, "Look! I can't do my job if you are going to keep looking over my shoulder." She went into a pout. We had apologies. I thought things were okay.

Clarice was preparing to accompany several of my voice students in a recital. Saturday afternoon, while she was practicing the piano accompaniments, she started banging on the piano, then got up and stomped around the room, screaming, "I can't play this!" The sudden noise sent me through the ceiling. I felt like I was being shot. Finally came her tears. She collapsed into my arms, crying, "I want to do everything right for you."

The next day, during my debut directing the choir at Saint Andrew, I kept missing cues. From her seat on the organ bench, Clarice had to prod me to get up at the right time to conduct the choral pieces. I felt awkward and out of place. Did we make a mistake taking this job? But the new job was not the culprit. Other forces, internal and external, were rushing in faster than we could fend them off.

CHAPTER 4

PREPARATION

The day after that numbing initiation at Saint Andrew, I flew to Kansas City on business for the ADM church music workshop. The 1996 workshop was to be at William Jewell College. I was program chair for the 1996 workshop, so I had to make a site visit and prepare a report at this year's (1995) workshop. Warren, the pastor friend who had administered the anointing ceremony for me two years earlier, met me at the airport and took me to our meeting. My findings during the site visit were to complicate our lives immeasurably in the next few weeks.

Warren had undergone a radical prostatectomy three years before. I waited until after our meeting was over, when I had his undivided attention in the privacy of his car, before broaching the subject of cancer and healing. He responded that he, too, had experienced the anointing of oil, laying on of hands, and concentrated prayer on his behalf. At the time of our conversation, he had tested negative for cancer. If nothing changed by his next checkup, he would be declared cancer-free. Even though I had now twice experienced the "healing oil," I privately doubted any direct link between his anointing and his clean bill of health.

While I was at Warren's house, Clarice called to report that we had a definite date for surgery: Wednesday, July 5. Dr. Shiller wanted to do it earlier, but he was going on vacation. July 5 would be his first day back on the job. Since prostate cancer usually grows very slowly, his urgency in wanting to speed toward the surgery disturbed me. I wondered if mine was growing faster than normal.

Back at home, regular business called. My private voice studio was full for the summer. My top high school student was preparing a full recital for the next Sunday, June 25. Joining her would be a former award-winning student who was currently at Indiana University; and Rosie Deal, a recent graduate of DePauw University. I had developed a strong bond with all three of these exceptionally talented young women, especially Rosie. After our last rehearsal, I told them that their recital was going to be my last musical production before going in for surgery. The shock and disbelief on their faces seared into my mind. I assured them that I would plan to return to limited teaching, at home, the week following the surgery. The joke was to be on me.

In the days leading up to the surgery, Clarice and I experienced a vitality and freedom in sex that led me to say, "If God had known how much fun sex was going to be, he probably would have chosen another means of propagating the species."

My birthday on June 27 played second fiddle to preparations for surgery.

[Journal entry, June 27, 1995. Birthday number fifty-four] Mother told me I was born at home. I don't believe Daddy was in the house. I was thirty days late. Mother went into labor. The nurse came. The doctor was on his way. The nurse coached her: "Now, give with this one, Mrs. Stegall. . . . Give with this one. . . . Don't give with *this* one!"

The doctor got there barely in time to catch me. He took one look and said, "Well, Mrs. Stegall, this is *not* a little baby." I weighed eleven pounds.

That's all I remember Mother telling me about my birth. Then, the year after I was married and was working on my doctorate at the University of Iowa, Mother told me more while we were sitting under the weeping willow tree in our backyard in Iowa City. She said I spent my first year in the crib. Mother's excuse was, "With Mamma there and me being sick, I just couldn't spend my time chasing you around."

I had exploded at her, "So *that's* why I grew up uncoordinated and overweight!"

But: *I am not what Mother did or did not do to me.*

I am who I let God make of me.

I will rejoice and be glad.

I had been saving my "gig" money (extra earnings) toward buying a new computer. When I realized the surgery was inevitable, I asked Clarice if we should save the money. She said, no, I had saved for the computer and we would need it to prepare materials for the music workshop. I did not ask twice. Because I wanted to work on the computer while I was recuperating, I made the decision and plunked down the money on Wednesday. I called it my "birthday present from me."

Thursday, June 29, was prescreening for the surgery. The nurse who took me through the paces was bright, cheerful, and attuned to my discomfort. One tech tried to draw blood. She got nothing. She tried the other arm. I started feeling weak and dizzy. The nurse took me around to one of the pre-op beds and told me to lie down. She sent the tech away and just talked with me for a few minutes. When she found out I was a voice teacher, she said, "I've always wanted to take lessons!" After chatting a while, she went about her other duties.

I looked around. This was the same room I would be in next week for surgery prep. Now it became a dress rehearsal for the real thing. People in adjoining alcoves waited to be wheeled into surgery. Nearby an anesthesiologist gave a patient his routine about what to expect.

Reality hit: *This is really happening, happening to me. That doctor is going to slice my abdomen from stem to sternum and take away my manhood. It will hurt. I will bleed. Something could go wrong. I could die. I'll never have sex again.*

Another tech came in. She was able to get blood. The nurse came back and went over the details of prep and post-op. She would be my surgical nurse. Her brightness was not superficial. I could read real compassion in her. Though I was full of anxiety, I felt strength coming from her.

At home encouraging calls and cards rolled in. One of the first callers was Vera Enz, a dear friend and fellow church musician from Edmund, Oklahoma. When she called I exclaimed, "Has this thing been on CNN?" Although we got much encouragement from friends far and near, our new church was silent. *They don't know me yet. However, Clarice has been there since February. It seems like someone would call.*

Another correspondence came from our attorney. He reminded us that we had never signed our living will declarations. We read through the documents that he so thoughtfully sent. We pondered the legalese as best we could, legalese that declared that, should our bodies wind up in a state that renders "sentient life" impossible, we would request only palliative care.

On Friday, June 30, I took the living will document down to the lawyer's office, got it all duly signed and notarized, then met Christopher Hollingsworth for lunch. Chris, talented, bright, and earnest, was to marry Rosie Deal in August. "My Rosie," one of the brightest lights in my teaching career, had gone on from high school to major in voice at DePauw University, where she had become a star. After graduating she returned to me for a few months of lessons. That had been the first time in my teaching career when I had been able to take the matured fruits of my early teaching and develop them even further.

Chris is the age of my older son. Rosie is the age of my daughter. Chris is academic. Rosie is a stage personality. Chris is a tenor. Rosie is a soprano. Tenor marrying soprano can be a lethal combination. It was time to meet Chris and give him encouragement. We had a rich exchange. When I revealed to him that I was fifty-four, he expressed surprise. "That's my dad's age, but somehow you seem a lot younger." That sealed it. He had my blessing!

That evening, five days before surgery, Maennerchor friends arranged a night with the boys at the Ale Emporium. It was supposed to be a gathering for spiritual support with several of the men who had been in the anointing ceremony two weeks earlier. At the Ale Emporium, multiple televisions blared a multitude of sporting events through the fog of cigarette smoke. Country music screamed from the PA system. Hundreds of patrons shouted to compete with the music and TV. I don't like crowds. I don't like noise. I don't like TV with my dinner. I don't like country music. I can't stand smoky rooms. I don't like beer.

The conversation, if one can call it that, turned to computers. I told the guys about the computer I had just bought. Suddenly they were all experts. Over the raucous din, they bombarded me with advice. "You don't want WordPerfect. You want Microsoft Word."

Finally I lost it. "Don't try to tell me what I want!" I yelled back. Thus went our two hours of spiritual consultation.

CHAPTER 5

SURGERY

On Saturday, July 1, I became the maid. The little apartment we had fixed up for Mumzy (Clarice's mother) when she came to live with us in 1988 was a cozy place on the ground level of our four-level house. It had a kitchen and a half bath. After Mumzy moved to a nursing home in February 1992, the apartment had reverted to cave status, inhabitable only by teenagers and dogs. I opened the windows, shampooed the carpets and furniture, and moved Mumzy's daybed back in. I hooked up the walkie-talkies we had bought for her. This room would be my campground until I could handle stairs.

On Sunday, July 2, Clarice and I presented a July Fourth musical program at Saint Andrew. This was my first time to sing at our new church. It was also the last time I would function professionally there until fall.

Monday, July 3, required the kinds of errands one does before leaving for vacation: fixing door locks, cleaning house, and so on. But first I had to judge a Shriners' choral competition. What I will do for a few bucks! A couple of the choirs could actually sing in tune. Afterward I took my living will declaration to Dr. Lukowski for his files. That evening Clarice and I went to hear the Indianapolis Symphony in their outdoor "Symphony on the Prairie" summer series. Downey Avenue Church had given me a packet of tickets as a farewell gift. It turned out to be a splendid evening, with real cannons on the *1812 Overture,* spectacular fireworks on *The Stars and Stripes Forever,* and a great excuse to cuddle on a hillside with my sweetheart.

We had been having as much sex as possible. This night turned out to be the last possible.

On Tuesday, July 4, my only independence was freeing myself of food. It was time to go on a liquid diet and take big glops of Dulcolax. My system had to be totally cleaned out. If the surgeon slipped and cut through the intestinal wall, and fecal material leaked into the abdominal cavity, peritonitis could set in. So Clarice fixed the most patriotic meal the diet would permit: red Jello for lunch and blue Jello for dinner. I figured the peritonitis scare was just a smokescreen. The real reason was to get me to thinking "sick." The liquid diet would make me so sick I would be glad to get to the hospital. We got more cards and calls offering prayers and support. The real cheater: I felt too lousy for sex.

On Wednesday, July 5, Operation Day, my dream of surprising the doc with a purified prostate evaporated when Dr. Shiller called in the morning to check in and answer any questions. I said, "What if you get in there and don't find any cancer?" He said they couldn't tell by eye. They had to wait for pathology to tell them. So out it comes anyhow.

I finished setting up the new computer that morning, just in time to leave for the hospital. Jeremy showed me how to use the word processor, and said, "Good luck. Can I have some lunch money?" That was pretty demonstrative for him at his current age of seventeen.

His behavior was a far cry from what it had been fourteen years before, when I had taken all three children camping in the Great Smokies while Clarice was away at a music workshop. The first day out, I had gotten such a sick headache that all I could do was lie in the tent and moan. While Jon and Joi, ages eleven and eight, stood around acting embarrassed, three-year-old Jeremy instinctively knew what to do. He lay down beside me and wrapped his arms around my neck. He comforted both of us and saved the camping trip from disaster.

Fasting for twenty-four hours heightened the senses. When we got to the hospital, my nose, usually dull, picked up the faintest hints of antiseptic, flowers, and cologne. Voices sounded like they were speaking into an ear trumpet. Five ministers, including Cyndi Alte, came to see me off. Three others, including my former pastor, Bryon Rose, and my current pastor, Nancy Howard, sent good wishes. George Keene, one of my Maennerchor friends, also came over; he even raced up I-65 from Kentucky to try to get there before I went under.

As I walked down the hall to yet another blood draw, an aide stopped me. "Are you Mr. Stegall?" She had come to tell me that the nurse who had done my prescreening had jury duty and would not be in today. She had called especially to give me the word. I couldn't believe it would make that much difference to a nurse whether she was there for one surgery or another. The nurse I did have was excellent.

She started an IV of Valium. Cyndi Alte, now a pastor, formerly a nurse, came in. I said to her, "I can't tell if this stuff is doing anything."

Cyndi chuckled. "Your eyes are rolling as you say that."

When the orderly came to roll me into surgery, I said, "Let me go to the bathroom first."

"Don't worry. They're going to put in a catheter anyway."

"But I want to do it one more time the real way."

That's the last I remember. No angel visitations. No opening skies. No long tunnel. No bright light. No seeing myself on the table. Just out.

When I gained consciousness my first words were, "Did they do the nerve sparing?"

The answer was no. The prostate turned out to be nearly full of malignancy (Gleason score of 7), with a small "positive margin," meaning there were some malignant cells on the surface. Dr. Shiller explained that it was too risky to try to spare the nerves. There was too much chance that malignant cells may be hiding under the nerves. He had biopsied the surrounding tissue and had removed the closest lymph nodes. No spreading of the cancer was detected. All this was abstract information to me. All I wanted was sleep.

They put me in a private room because no double rooms were available. I asked if insurance would cover the private room. Yes, it would, but only until a semiprivate room became available. "What's the difference in cost?"

"Twenty dollars a day." It was worth paying the difference to get to stay where I was.

The next day several of my Maennerchor friends came by. With their cumulative visits, I was in conversation probably two hours. That was an hour and fifty minutes too much.

By the second day, the pain reared its head. Mary Alice, known as "M. A.," was the nurse on duty. Once, while she was in the room, I accidentally jerked the catheter. Pain shot through my abdomen. I sobbed and shook, unable to control the abdomen. I tried to talk, but no words would come out. I finally got her to hand me my little journal pad. I wrote on it, "I feel so lonesome and helpless."

M. A. held my hand firmly, talking quietly. "Think of a place you would like to be. A favorite vacation place, maybe."

I managed to answer: "My daughter is coming home. My son is getting married." In a minute or so, I was calm enough to let go of her hand. She and the other staff were outstanding. I came to realize that the nursing staff is more important to a surgery patient's recovery than is the surgeon, who can collect his check and go home.

Every first was a threat: emptying the catheter bag, changing the leg bag, walking with help, walking alone, being alone. The sense of loss was overwhelming. I cried more than I had since the first time I saw *Bambi*.

I scrupulously avoided looking at my abdomen when I went to the bathroom. It was bad enough to think of being stapled like a piece of furniture upholstery. But my eyes slipped up once and caught a glimpse in the mirror of metallic teeth gleaming at me. I nearly passed out. I thought of Dr. Zhivago, when he staggered into Lara's house after wandering the wastelands, with ice crusted on his beard, his eyes red and sunken, then looked at himself in the mirror. The next time I looked at the incision, it looked like a zipper. I remembered what Mother said after her gall bladder surgery: "Women should be made with a zipper."

The nurses told me they could release me from the hospital after I had a bowel movement. The bowels shut down during surgery, so they have to make sure the bowels get jump-started before they let you go. I tried, but even the slightest pressure sent spasms of pain through the abdomen. In one attempt, just getting to the bathroom was more than I could handle. As I sat on the toilet gazing at the bare wall and sobbing, again "I to the hills lift up mine eyes," to Jean Berger's music, ran through my head.

I remembered Daddy's talking about the proper punctuation for that verse: "I lift up my eyes to the hills. *Period.* From whence comes my help?

Question mark. My help comes from the Lord, who made heaven and earth! *Exclamation point.*" The punctuation brought comfort. I could see no hills. All I saw was a white wall with an emergency chain hanging on it. The help comes not from the hills, but from God!

On Saturday Dr. Shiller dropped in. He said everything looked good and that I could go home when I was ready. I asked if I could stay until Sunday so Clarice would not have to bother with me while she was taking care of the music at church on Sunday. He agreed. That was better treatment than new mothers are getting now.

On Sunday morning the syndicated story program *Rabbit Ears Radio* came over National Public Radio, presenting Hans Christian Andersen's "The Snow Princess." The Snow Princess freezes the boy Kay into an ice statue. When his friend Gerda finds him, she weeps over him. Her hot tears melt the ice, freeing Kay. The two children break into victorious laughter. As long as they laugh, the Snow Princess cannot work magic on them.[10]

The story delivered a special message. In my half-sleeping state, I realized: tears and laughter, *in that order,* bring healing.

> I wept
> until there were no more tears
> I hurt
> until I was numb
> I feared
> until I was paralyzed
> I worried
> until I was sick
>
> Then I laughed
> Laughter vibrated through my muscles
> releasing my stiff body
> Laughter vibrated through my soul
> replenishing my tears
>
> Having laughed
> I was released
> from fear
> and worry

Having laughed
I could feel again
I could move again
Having laughed
I could hurt again
I could weep again
Having laughed
My soul was full again
My soul was well again[11]

CHAPTER 6

ON MY OWN

Once home, I was on my own while Clarice and Jeremy were at work. One morning, lying in bed while Clarice got ready to go to work, I became overwhelmed with emotion, bursting out with, "I can't believe that you can love me so much."

Clarice acted self-conscious when I told anyone how fantastic she was. "Don't make me a saint," she admonished. Not to worry. Whenever I got ready to pronounce the grace of beatification, something would happen to bring us back to earth. Something really important—something that is a watershed in a person's life—something like leaving shoes where someone could trip over them.

The time alone was essential for building up strength and working on the next goal: plans for the 1996 workshop would not wait. When this year's workshop convened at St. Olaf University, in Northfield, Minnesota, I had to have the basic plans ready for the next year. Eleven days after my release from the hospital, I was to meet with the ADM president, president-elect, and our professional staff to lay the groundwork for the next year.

By the second day at home, I was dragging myself down the half flight of stairs to the basement, where the new computer waited, to start putting together schedules so they would be ready for the July 20 meeting.

To meet that deadline, we pushed up the dates for taking out staples and removing the catheter. Somehow "getting staples out" sounds more drastic than does "getting stitches out." I still avoided looking at the incision. They didn't bother Clarice at all. She said, "What a neat job!" So I gave Clarice the job of examining the incision for signs of inflammation.

The day I wanted to skip came too soon. When Dr. Shiller's nurse saw the incision, she exclaimed, "Oh, that's the most beautiful incision I've ever seen!"

So this is what gives you a thrill, I thought. *Let's just get on with it.*

But she wanted to take the easy approach. She laid me out on the table like a slab of beef. "This little instrument acts just like a regular staple remover. I'll start at the top. I go real slow and easy."

"Don't tell me. Just do it."

She was compulsive. "There's one . . . two . . . three . . . We're doing real good."

The first two or three were just little pricks. *This won't be so bad.* I was foolish. Again.

"Now it is going to get a little more tender." She was right. It seemed like she had removed a couple dozen staples.

Should be over soon.

She had to give me a progress report. "We're doing great. We're almost half done."

Half done? That did it. I had to stop. I had gone through Lamaze childbirth classes with Clarice. I had practiced relaxation breathing with her and with all my voice students since then. Every day, thirty times a week, relaxation breathing. Now when I needed it, I couldn't make it work.

The nurse left. Dr. Shiller came in. Zip-zip-zip, he had them out. Now I could breathe without those things pulling on the skin every time the abdomen expanded.

I thought I was strong enough to teach, so I set up some lessons on each of two days at home. After two hours I was ready for bed. I canceled the next day's schedule.

That weekend Joi was to come home from Oklahoma. She had been away for two years. Her devotion to school and work had even prevented her from coming home for holidays during the past year. We were ecstatic at her decision to return to Indianapolis. She planned to go back to work at the veterinary clinic where she had worked before going to Oklahoma, and enroll in school here. Jeremy flew to Oklahoma to help her pack and to share the driving. On Saturday they started out from Stillwater, pulling the largest trailer that U-Haul had.

Saturday night Joi called. "Dad, the transmission on my car gave out near Springfield, Missouri. We got a tow truck to take the car and trailer directly to the local U-Haul office. The tow truck driver gave us a ride to a motel nearby. Jeremy and I will go back in the morning to rent a truck, then tow the car home." That meant that Jeremy would have to single-handedly unload the trailer and load the truck. He's a strong, strapping young man, but I ached to think of his doing that task, alone, in the July heat.

I said: "That's good thinking! But how are you going to pay for it?"

"Maybe you could help us out?" What a surprise request.

Sunday evening, while we were waiting for Joi and Jeremy, we heard a sound like lightning striking in our backyard. Our lights all went out. We looked out the back window to see that the power lines feeding the house were on fire. I immediately called 911. Within minutes the rescue squad, firefighters, and police were swarming over our yard. One of the major wires had by now burned in two, and, still shooting sparks, dangled within inches of our shrubs. I, who was still supposed to be "conserving my strength," tromped, in my pajamas, around the yard with the authorities. They discovered the source: a burned-out transformer. Power company workers labored until late into the night to repair the damage.

That same Sunday evening, Joi and Jeremy arrived, driving a truck large enough to move a household and towing her crippled '85 Honda. Joi came to the door carrying her cat, innocently named Rebekkah. The name is the only innocent characteristic of that cat. Prince, eighty-five pounds of Great Dane and yellow Labrador, was our Shakespearian pet: he loved "not wisely but too well." Prince jumped up to see what Joi was holding in her arms. Rebekkah, spying the fiercest-looking creature she had ever seen, panicked. She tried to claw out of Joi's arms, biting her in the process. Joi, animalwise, washed out the wound with peroxide and forgot about it.

Monday morning I called several places about repairing the transmission on Joi's car. Most of the cost estimates were more than her car was worth. If I went into detail here, a major national company might sue me for libel. Suffice it to say that the transmission adventure (not even including the electrical fire and Joi's cat bite, about which more was to come) one week after leaving the hospital, sucked up my residual physical and emotional energy. Joi's car was to languish in a back lot at the transmission place for six weeks.

By Monday Joi's cat bite became inflamed. She was smart enough to take herself to see Dr. Lukowski. He treated the wound and drew a ring around the outside of the inflamed area. He instructed her that if the inflammation spread beyond the marked boundary, she would need to go to the hospital.

Tuesday evening Dr. Shiller's urology group convened a new prostate cancer support group. Clarice and I decided to go. I felt like an old man, hanging on to her arm to steady myself as we walked. Dr. Shiller's bug eyes popped out three feet when he saw me shuffling down the hallway toward him. I looked around at the thirty or so men and various wives, and said to Dr. Shiller: "It looks like I'm not only the newest patient here but also the youngest! Most of these guys are ten to twenty years older than I am."

The presenter, however, was younger than I was—also a doctor. He was a fifty-two-year-old urologist in practice with Dr. Shiller. He had, within the past year, undergone the same surgery as I. He had also had radiation. He confessed that being a doctor did not make it any easier to handle treatment and recovery. He had to deal with impotence, incontinence, depression—all the same consequences many men there had faced or would face. *Maybe my feeling rotten doesn't really mean that I'm a wimp. Maybe I'm just normal.*

Wednesday, exactly a week after the staples episode and one day before I was to fly to St. Olaf, the catheter had to come out. I dreaded this even more than the staples. There is something about having a tube pulled out from the most sensitive orifice of my body that gave me the willies. Perhaps, however, a flexible plastic tube is an improvement over the Nile reeds used by the ancient Egyptians.

After a few days, I had gotten accustomed to the catheter. The large Foley bag took care of one problem: I did not have to get up to go to the bathroom in the night. When I saw how much urine accumulated in one night, I marveled that the bladder did not burst or fill up the entire abdomen under normal use. The only problem I ever had was the night I forgot to close the emptying tube, awakening to a floor covered with a quart or so of urine.

One of my friends told me his catheter was inserted while he was fully conscious; then he had to take it out himself. I knew enough anatomy to understand how it worked. There were actually two little tubes in one sheath. One tube drained the bladder. The other tube had an inflatable bulb on the inside end. The technician would run water up the tube to fill the bulb, then would seal the outside end. The little bulb created a stopper to keep the catheter from accidentally pulling out. To remove it, all you had to do was open the end, let the water drain out, and pull.

No way. I not only dreaded the process of pulling it out but also the new adjustment to wearing Depends while one muscle learned to do the job of three.[12]

George Keene was my taxi this time so Clarice would not have to get off of work again. A new nurse greeted me. Again I had to lie down on the table and pull my pants down. By this stage of my medical adventure, I didn't care very much anymore.

I closed my eyes and tried to relax. This nurse did not give me a play-by-play. Suddenly I felt my insides being pulled out through the smallest possible opening. I instinctively grabbed at the intruding hand. She was faster than I was. It was over.

She brought me a small supply of Depends and left the room. Now was the time to use another gem I had picked up in Lamaze classes. Kegel exercises strengthen the sphincter muscles that control urination and, in women, strengthen the vaginal sling muscles. Back when we had practiced Kegeling in Lamaze classes, we were strengthening the same muscles that singers need for deep breath support. My college voice teacher called it the "dime exercise." When she wanted me to reach for deeper breath support while singing, she would sing out, "Grip that dime, boy, grip that dime!"

I grabbed the Kegel position and stood up. *Whoosh.* The pad was full. Sat down. Unloaded and reloaded. *Whoosh.* At this rate I would use up a whole bag of diapers before I got home. I reloaded again. My teacher's voice sprang into my head: "Grip that dime, boy, grip that dime!" I gripped tighter. Got up slowly. No *whoosh.* Just a little drip.

Finding my way out to the receptionist to schedule my next appointment, I felt dizzy. "Do you need to sit down?" she asked. I shook my head but she did not believe me. The nurse led me back to the examining room and got me a cola. In a few minutes, I was able to stumble out to the waiting room where George was waiting, patient as Buddha.

That night I got out one of the heavy-duty Depends. This one fit around like a real diaper. Only babies, old people, and mentally incompetent people had to use them. But now I, a properly housebroken adult, faced infant dependency.

That same day, Wednesday, Joi's cat bite infection got out of control. She was to spend the next two days in the hospital on an IV-controlled antibiotic.

On Thursday it was time to get on a plane bound for St. Olaf University in Northfield, Minnesota, to take care of music workshop business.

CHAPTER 7

NORTHFIELD, MINNESOTA

Clarice did not fly to Minnesota with me. Because I had to get to St. Olaf two days ahead of the workshop, she opted to work those days and fly out on Saturday. Besides, now she had a sick daughter to take care of. But I was not forsaken. The Mamma of all Mammas rode with me. Freida Armstrong was the administrative assistant for ADM from the church headquarters in Indianapolis. She and Clarice had arranged for wheelchair and shuttle service in the airports. I kept my eye out for all the restroom locations, because I had to change pads about every hour. Freida would have fed me a bottle and pureed my food if I had let her. She has never met a stranger. She got me acquainted with everyone in the airport. And the system worked. We made all our connections. By 2:00 PM I was in the hotel in Northfield, Minnesota, where the planning council would stay until the workshop opened.

Neither body nor psyche was prepared for the business we confronted in our first mini-council meeting Thursday evening. My report on the site visit in Kansas City pointed out many trouble spots regarding the size of meeting rooms, walking distances, hills, handicapped accessibility, and so on. All present concurred that we would have to find another location for 1996. Although we usually choose our locations two or three years ahead, I now had three days to find a new site for the next year. In between runs to the bathroom, I spent several hours calling colleges, finally finding a couple that could accommodate our schedule.

Freida ordered a wheelchair for me to use during the workshop. It arrived just before lunch on Friday. The council immediately dubbed it the "Chalicemobile," after the Church chalice and cross symbol. I said, "No, thank you, I'll walk." A flight of twenty-four steps stood between our residence hall and the dining hall. June, who had, along with Warren, anointed me for healing two years earlier, walked up the steps with me, holding my hand. June is a round, grandmotherly ordained minister. I felt very comfortable telling her all about the surgery as we walked. By the top of the steps, I was out of breath and dizzy.

At lunch we had a great reunion with the full council. The first major debate concerned the critical question as to whether I would ride the wheelchair or walk on the campus tour. Freida prevailed. I rode. Riding in the wheelchair gave me a firsthand perspective on the limitations, the difference, the dependence of a person who would have to live in a wheelchair.

During the first full council meeting Friday afternoon, I became dizzy. My stomach started cramping. I thought I could just lie down on the floor, but as I knelt down, I felt extremely dizzy. Freida put me in the wheelchair and wheeled me around the corner to a room with a bed. Left alone, I started shaking, sobbing, and hyperventilating. I needed my sweetie. I forced myself to take slow, deep breaths. A minute or so later, I was relaxed enough to sleep.

[Dream] "Carmen" had taken up with "Rob Starling." She hinted that she was going to marry him. She seemed sly, crafty, almost gleeful in telling me. This man seemed to own Chimney Rock. The man wanted me to sign over my furniture refinishing business to him. After all, he reasoned, I wasn't doing anything with it. He could move the business to Chimney Rock and make it prosper for him and Carmen. I thought, "Oh, why not?" It's not doing me any good."

[Observation] "Carmen" was a young woman toward whom I had felt some sexual attraction. Chimney Rock is a real place in the Blue Ridge Mountains, where a huge rock "chimney" protrudes out of the side of the mountain. Its resemblance to an erect penis is obvious.

Daddy was a master furniture builder, refinisher, and restorer. That is the one role in which I saw him as traditionally masculine: proud, competent, and in control. His gift with wood is the role that I wish I could emulate. The dream was asking me to give up my masculinity.

People arriving early for the workshop had dinner on Friday evening at the Tavern, in "downtown" Northfield. I sat with a lively table of party animals, including longtime friend Katrina, a PhD psychologist. Brad, our official photographer, wanted a cozy picture of Katrina and me. As we snuggled cheek to cheek, I murmured in her ear, "It's okay. I'm perfectly safe."

Still posing, she answered, "There are ways around that, you know." She knew someone who used the pump implant. "We'll get a threesome with Clarice and talk about it."

Having to push a button to pump up an erection did not appeal to me. Certainly having another surgery was out of the question. I thought a vacuum tube might be okay. I'd find out about that in due time.

By Sunday the site for our next workshop became the primary item on the council agenda. I gave my report, and then said: "I'm going to do something unprecedented. I am going to move that the council reject my report and find another location for 1996." We debated and fielded inquiries for three days. The council members were extraordinarily considerate of my limitations. Yet they needed answers that only I could give. I had to force myself just to keep up with the discussion, much less to gather data and make reasonable recommendations.

After three days of sometimes-divisive debate, the Council voted overwhelmingly to change the 1996 site to the University of Tulsa. That decision would precipitate many more hours of work during and after the workshop. It also meant extra work reconciling feelings that were injured during the debate.

Besides the public duties, I set three private goals for the week: to be free of the "Chalicemobile" wheelchair, to sleep without Depends, and to make love to my wife. I sometimes used the "Chalicemobile" as a walker, or simply as a luggage buggy. Well-meaning ladies would chide me, "You get in that chair and ride!" But I knew I had to walk to regain strength if

I was to be completely free of the chair by the end of the workshop. By Tuesday I began trying stairs. Tuesday night Clarice and I engaged in real lovemaking for the first time since July 3. I did not know if I could expose myself to her touch. She just giggled: "You're bald as a billiard ball." We were both then at ease. Every touch was erotic, healing, and spiritual. There is this to be said about unfulfilled passion: It can keep going forever. That night I slept without Depends for the first time.

By long-standing tradition, the workshop closed with the entire gathering of 250 musicians joining hands in a big circle singing Peter Lutkin's "The Lord Bless You and Keep You." That tradition had been established many years previously by Weston Noble, conductor of the famed Nordic Choir of Luther College.

After a final council meeting the next morning, Clarice and I headed home. While waiting for our flight from the Minneapolis airport, I felt the pressure in my bladder that said, "I need to urinate." That was the first time I had felt that pressure since the surgery. Previously it would just start dribbling. *Okay. Those Kegel exercises we learned in Lamaze classes are paying off! The one remaining sphincter muscle is starting to work.*

CHAPTER 8

HOME AND TO WORK

fter taking all of July off from teaching, I had a dream that told me I was ready to resume teaching.

[Dream] An attractive young woman in her early twenties worked as a clerk but wanted to be a singer. She had sharp, clean features and a triangular jaw with sharp points at the chin and the back of the jaw. I asked her to sing something for me. She sang, to a clearly defined melody:

"Turn   loose   from   your   gold- en   pre- ten- ses"
"SOL   mi   re   do   SOL SOL FI   LA   SOL"

The voice was a warm, rich mezzo-soprano, but her jaw and tongue were tense and quivering. I suggested that she not try to stretch the jaw so much in the mid-voice; that, believe it or not, it would take a lot of pressure off the voice.

[Observation] I often dream melodies. For several years I carefully notated most of them when I woke up. Sometimes, like this one, the dream supplies words as well as tune. Just such a person did, indeed, come to my studio for lessons about a year later.

After that dream I decided it was time to get back to work! Measuring my stamina by my daily walk, I realized that, initially, I would give out after walking a hundred yards. After teaching for four hours, I was sobbing with exhaustion. Meanwhile, Clarice returned to work. The workshop had not been a vacation for her. Now she had to take care of me and work. She had ample reason for being strung out.

I had a contract with my fitness gym to tell stories to their day camp children. The Thursday after returning from St. Olaf was my first "gig" since the surgery. I was unprepared, technically and emotionally. Programs for preschoolers always require extra preparation. I don't do them as well as those for older children, and I don't enjoy them as much. And now the energy was near zero. But I showed up at the appointed time. The children arrived. I went through an action story and game with them. Energy began stirring through my body. At the end of the program, a little girl ran back to tell me I was a good storyteller.

The older children came in. A number of them had their own agendas. Counselors threatened. It never does any good. It is the *story* that gets them. One of the boys yelled, "Tell the 'Moldy' story."

The "Moldy" story. It is always the fifth-and-sixth-grade boys who ask for it. I call it "The Banana in the Desk," a true story that happened to me in first grade. That banana stayed in the desk for a week, rotting and molding. Then Mrs. Davis made me clean it out in full view of the class. The boys love calling me "Moldy" for several days after every time I tell it.

"I told it last time."

"Well, tell it for the ones who didn't hear it last time."

So here goes—again. I love telling it, but this time it felt stale. The energy generated with the younger children was spent out. I felt drained and shaky by the time we finished.

Phil had been widowed in 1992. He had remarried in 1994 to Janean, a widowed family friend. They both sang in my church choir. The entire community had rejoiced in the budding romance. I had put together a choir of friends and family from around the country to sing for their wedding. Phil had lived with epilepsy for many years. I had witnessed him going into petit mal seizures, when he would just fog out for a minute, then come back in where he had left off. On Monday, July 31, he went to work at the LaRue D. Carter Hospital Library, where he had been a psychiatric reference librarian for many years. He had a grand mal seizure, went into cardiac arrest, and was dead in minutes.

On Friday, August 4, we laid Phil to rest. He was fifty-seven. His whole family, plus his new wife's family and the entire community, came. We could hardly get a seat in the church for the funeral.

Phil was a quiet man who loved doing things for people. He told me once that when people would come into his library, looking for a reference for "a friend," he would get the references, then talk with them about the "friend's" concern. He felt he had directed people to get help who may not have sought it otherwise.

His organist brother, who had played for Phil and Janean's wedding just a year earlier, played for the funeral. Just as it had been for the wedding, the church overflowed for the funeral.

Phil's youngest daughter was a high school classmate of Rosie Deal's. The next day was Rosie's wedding. I felt that I had to attend the wedding. I planned my arrival for five minutes before the ceremony, sitting at the back so I could leave if I had to. Afterward I wrote a letter to the newlyweds.

Dear Rosie and Chris:

Today I was part of a step in the great spiral of life. A wedding is a community celebration. And what a celebration this one was! At least four, maybe five generations, including a number of young children and babies, all came. There were people of all shapes, ages, and races. There were the elegant and the plain. A young woman, resplendent in her usual beauty, had just said farewell to her father the day before. But there she was, along with others of your high school friends. And then there were the college friends, including two skilled young soloists who have not suffered enough to comprehend, totally, what they were singing. That is part of the proper order.

I believe we are endowed by our Creator with a genetic amnesia. The younger generation forgets, genetically, what their parents and grandparents back to antiquity knew. If a new generation were to approach marriage and childbearing fully knowing what lay in store, civilization would come to a screeching halt.

We of the "wiser" generation complain, "We can't tell them a thing!" But therein lies our hope, for you must do as we did and continue to do. You must learn to live by living.

Your marriage is especially poignant to me for several reasons. You are about the ages of my two older children, one of whom is to be married in two weeks. I have known Rosie for eight years. Because I have moved a lot (in my first twelve years, I lived in six different towns), this is the first time in my professional life that I have been able to see the development of a brilliant young singer through high school, college, and on to the beginning of a career and marriage. Finally, there is who you are: Rosemary and Christopher, two gifted, intelligent young people who appear to adore each other.

I offer you my testimony that it can get even better. That genetic amnesia serves another purpose: You cannot, at this point, anticipate the depths, heights, and riches of a love that has weathered and survived. But with God's help, you can partake. Call me in twenty-five years and let me know.

CHAPTER 9

ANNIVERSARY AND WEDDING

Yet other events rushed in: a reunion with Lyle and Linda, Clarice's brother and sister-in-law; our twenty-seventh wedding anniversary; our son Jon's wedding. Lyle had come from California to visit us in Indianapolis only once, three years earlier, in January 1992, just before Mumzy went to the nursing home.

On their way to the wedding, Lyle and Linda flew to Indianapolis from their home in California so he could see his mother. I took Lyle over to the nursing home. Lyle was not prepared for what he would find. Pearl Williams—Lyle and Clarice's mother, my "Mumzy," a hardworking woman who proudly wore the mantle of "housewife," who taught Sunday school, who took over the church treasurer position when her husband died, who was an active volunteer for "the old folks" until she was well into her eighties, and who was an eloquent public speaker—was now shriveled up in a wheelchair, nearly deaf, blind in her left eye (yet 20/40 in the right!). We had to strain to carry on the most rudimentary conversation.

I wheeled Mumzy out into the sunroom, and stayed out of her line of sight while Lyle tried to visit with her. Lyle, gregarious charmer, fluent preacher, accomplished gospel singer, looked toward me helplessly. "What do I do?" he pleaded.

"Sing to her. She likes 'Just as I Am,' 'Amazing Grace,' and 'Blessed Assurance.'"

Lyle gave it the old college try. He has a beautiful untrained voice that I with all my years of training can only envy. But he stumbled around, finally just telling her he loved her and giving her a kiss.

"I don't know how you do it," Lyle said to us. I remembered that when my mother had to go to nursing care, my brother Joel had been the one to take care of her.

"It's just our turn," I answered. We had given her permission to "go home" whenever she was ready. We all prayed that God would take her.

The next day Lyle, Linda, Clarice, and I piled into our rental compact car (remember the transmission? We were still waiting for Joi's car to get out of hock.) and headed toward North Carolina for Jon's wedding. We went out of our way to see longtime friends Bill and Joan Trathen, who had opened a bed and breakfast in Mountain City, Tennessee, right across the state line from North Carolina. Dr. Bill Trathen was the obstetrician who had delivered Jeremy. His wife, Joan, and daughter, Loren, had sung in the community chorus I started in Boone. We had been in a gourmet club with them.

Now in early retirement as gentleman farmer and gracious host, Bill easily recalled to Clarice the smallest details of Jeremy's delivery. "He about scared the life out of me. He had a fetal heartbeat of one hundred. Every time you contracted, his heartbeat went down. We prepped for a 'section. But when we got into delivery, I said, 'Try pushing, and let's see what happens.' Out he came." Bill had delivered multitudes of babies. Yet his recall after almost eighteen years was as specific as if he were reading off his medical chart.

It was August 17, our twenty-seventh wedding anniversary. Lyle and Linda told us this overnight was on them, their anniversary gift to us. Clarice and I tried to make love. Pleasuring was wonderful, but tonight I got built up with nowhere to go. Several times I had been able to enjoy the journey without worrying about rushing to the destination, but this time I felt so restless, I couldn't let go of Clarice and could not calm down.

I went to the bathroom after she had settled down to sleep. I stimulated myself and felt the surge of orgasm. I could not believe it! No erection. No ejaculation. But still—the sensation of orgasm.

The next night I told Clarice about it. She praised me like a mother praising her child for finishing his spinach. I tried to show her how to do it. It just would not work the second time.

Jon and Jamie's wedding was in a Baptist church far out in the country north of Charlotte, North Carolina. We need ceremony. We need rituals. We need excuses to gather friends and family from afar. Jon and Jamie were married two days after our wedding anniversary. They headed to the Outer Banks for their honeymoon, the same place Clarice and I had gone for our honeymoon in 1968.

The wedding afforded us a chance to visit with my brother, Joel, for the first time in over a year. We almost always make it a point to go off somewhere together so we can talk uninterrupted. The best we could manage this time was a brisk walk along a busy highway in front of our hotel. I have looked up to him since as far back as I can remember. This time, I realized, *he* was the one needing instruction. My cancer makes him face his own vulnerability. Statistically, my getting it makes him, his son, and my birth son high risks for the disease (Jon is adopted, and Asian, putting him at low risk for cancer). I was surprised at how freely I could converse with my brother about such intimate matters as impotence and incontinence.

CHAPTER 10

TO PROSTHETIZE OR NOT?

O n my next visit to Dr. Shiller for a follow-up PSA, I picked up flyers touting products promising the pretense of potency. Several were implants that required surgery. The Malleable, a "semirigid rod prosthesis," produces a "permanent erection that can be positioned close to the body during everyday activities." The flyer showed pictures of the Malleable in action and inaction. You just reach down and bend it up when you are ready. No waiting. I guess when you want to pee, you can sight it in any direction and let fly ("Look Ma, no hands"). The Inflatable "is implanted entirely within the body. When the man wants an erection, he transfers fluid to the cylinders from the reservoir by squeezing the pump (positioned in the scrotum) several times." The Hydroflex Self-Contained Penile Prosthesis has two pumps at the tip of the penis, for inflation and deflation. The vacuum pump creates an erection by drawing blood into the penis. It requires no surgery. If it could get the results on me that it showed on that man in the drawing, it would be worth the price.

One of my friends had tried it. "It works," he said. "You just have to watch out when you clamp the rubber bands around the base of the penis to keep up the erection. You can get them tangled in the pubic hair." I wondered if you could get gangrene. Nonetheless I asked Dr. Shiller to set up an appointment with the sales representative. If insurance would cover it, I might try it.

At that time Viagra and its offshoots were not in the picture. Even if it were, I would have been a poor candidate. Viagra is good for men who have erectile dysfunction, but does not create sexual desire or sexual function.

While we waited for the insurance company to deliver a verdict on the "medical necessity" of an erection device, there finally came the night when Clarice and I achieved, without benefit of mechanical aid, mutual orgasm. We were both overwhelmed. We lay in each other's arms, sobbing, for a long time.

It had only been in the past year that, in response to her questions, I had confessed that about every fourth female I saw turned me on. When she shook her head in mock disbelief, I protested: "I don't think about sex all the time. Sometimes I can go a whole hour without thinking about it." She already knew the essential fact that I have never had sex with anyone other than my wife. Since the surgery the sexual urgency had waned. But for now we could still awaken the sensations. But for how long? That was the question.

"I'm not going to talk with you unless you smile." The cocksure young man in a dark blue suit, white shirt, and red tie led me down the hallway where he was to demonstrate the vacuum pump.

Why should you expect me to smile? I haven't had lunch. I've waited an hour for you. You look like the kind of guy who will take on all the women you can get your hands on. And you're showing me something that is at best inconvenient, at worst humiliating. Why should I smile? I can no longer do what once was embarrassingly easy. Now I have to reveal my inadequacies to this Adonis. Could the company not line up a salesman who acted like he had some idea of the trauma his customers faced?

When he finished his presentation, he said, "All right, now let's drop your pants and we will see how you can make it work."

No way. What is this guy? "Let me take it home to try it."

"This is a demonstrator. You'll have to go to Eastside Prescription Shop to get the model you want. If you don't try it out here, you won't know which model you want."

"I'll take that risk."

Back home I told Clarice the whole story. She said: "It's completely up to you if you want to get it. But don't do it for my sake. You love me.

That's all I care about." She then showed me a story she had recently clipped from an Ann Landers column:

> A man went to his doctor for a cure for his impotence. The doctor outlined one treatment after another, with ever-increasing price tags. Finally he described an operation that would be guaranteed successful. It would cost $10,000. The man said, "Let me talk it over with my wife."
>
> The next day he returned to the doctor. The doctor asked, "Well, what did your wife say about the operation?"
>
> "She said she would rather have a new kitchen."[13]

Figuring I had nothing to lose, once my insurance company gave approval for the medical necessity of the vacuum pump, I ordered one of the devices. The instructions say to "practice with it for at least five days before putting it to use." So I practiced. Twice. No go. Not only was it uncomfortable, but it would spoil any romance we might cook up. It would take so long to get any action that we both would lose interest. It could be a turn-off for Clarice. Most likely she would take a look at the contraption and break out laughing.

The vacuum pump, all $450 worth of it, went to live in the closet for good. Eventually I put it on the "give and take" table at my support group meeting with a sign, "Never fired in anger." It disappeared in ten minutes.

About this time I decided to experiment with "flying without a net"—using no Depends. I went forty-two hours without a mishap. Just one squirt on Saturday. Several times I went to the gym to work out with no Depends. Even shooting baskets, running, jumping.

A friend had a prostatectomy three years before I did, when he was sixty-two. He also had radiation and chemotherapy. He was currently using DES, an estrogen product, to control the cancer growth. He had not regained continence in three years. He told me he was still using four Depends a day. I thought: "I can't complain. I really have it easy."

CHAPTER 11

EMOTIONAL FALLOUT

F inancial concerns, swimming about under the surface, popped their heads out of the water periodically. We had missed a month of my income. We knew the medical bills would be astronomical and did not know just how much insurance would pay. But the most persistent, and nettlesome, worry was that I may have to go into extended convalescence—or die. My family is not financially prepared for the loss of my income. I lay awake nights fretting about it.

Clarice was my strongest emotional support. As we moved into the fall, she began to fall apart. She bore several major burdens in addition to mine. Her mother lay in a nursing home, unable to speak or do anything for herself. When Clarice visited the nursing home, fear gripped her: "Will I end up like this?" Our younger son's senior year in high school lurked as a dark cloud. We knew the chances of his passing enough classes to graduate were slim. Even if he did graduate, what would he do then? Our daughter, recently returned from two years away from home, revealed that her stay in Oklahoma had not been a happy one. As a result she had become deeply depressed and near-anorexic.

Because of my own depression and fatigue, I was not able to give my wife, daughter, and son the support I knew they needed.

A major factor in Clarice's depression related to our new church music positions. She is an organist, an exceptionally gifted organist. Only once since leaving graduate school has she had a really fine organ to play on. At our new church, the organ, a grand 40-rank 1936 Kilgen, was literally in pieces, with pipes on the floor, in the choir room, in the balcony, in the halls, in the chapel. A couple of years before we came to Saint Andrew, the church had contracted a couple of builders to restore the organ. The builders had dismantled the instrument, then skipped town with the money they had demanded up front. Now the church was out half of its organ fund, what little work had been done was totally botched, and the organ repair committee could not come to a decision about what to do. The only thing that seemed conclusive was that they were determined to do the job using only the remaining money they still had from the old fund. Clarice dreaded practicing and playing on the few operable ranks.

She also had grown so accustomed to directing her own choir that it was difficult for her to become "just the organist."

On occasion our responses to the strain teetered toward the bizarre. One Saturday we went for an afternoon of shopping and a movie at Circle Center Mall, the new downtown shopping extravaganza. Indianapolis finally had a Nordstrom's, famous for customer service. Clarice wanted to look for shoes at Nordstrom's. She has been on a life-long quest for shoes that fit her ice-skate skinny feet. When we got to the store, we saw dozens of clerks scurrying about, bringing out piles of pricey shoes for hoards of customers. Clarice stood rooted in one place. "What am I doing here? I feel overwhelmed. I don't belong in a store like this. They don't care if they can fit me. I couldn't afford it if I could find a fit." A clerk came up and offered assistance. To my astonishment she turned him away. As he left, though, she muttered, "Maybe if I sit down and look pathetic, somebody might come."

I ventured, "Maybe you should try another store."

She started sobbing. "Fat help you are."

She finally spotted a clerk who had waited on her when he worked for another store. He fitted her with a nice pair of pumps.

We headed upstairs to the theater. In the movie queue, a woman asked me for the time. My tongue got tangled. It was 2:10, but I said, "10:05," then tried twice more before finally getting out the right time, creating much amusement among the people who were standing in line. When ordering the tickets, I could not say the name of the movie, *How to Make an American Quilt.* The consonants came out all slurred. I wanted to turn around and say: "Look, folks, I do know how to talk. I even teach English diction!" But they would probably think I was drunk.

CHAPTER 12

RADIATION

If a man has no prostate gland, he should secrete no PSA. The highest "safe" tolerance is a level of 1.0 ng/ml, though ideally it should be 0.00 ng/ml. A test in October read 0.6. Dr. Shiller was not pleased, but was not alarmed. He said if it was significantly higher at the next test, "We'll radiate you." I felt safe from that prospect. After all, he had gotten it all, hadn't he? He had a moral duty to give me the potential bad news: "Remember, we had a positive margin." No, I did not remember, though no doubt he had told me. *Positive margin* means that some bad cells were on the surface. Even though the surrounding tissues biopsied negative, there could be some residual malignant cells. So he immediately took another PSA draw. This one read 3.0. Now it was time to see the radiologist.

[Dream] I saw a road with cartoonlike people and cars on it. The road went straight up and down hills. There were no curves. A voice came out of the sky, "I thought faith was such that, as you lived longer, the hills would level out so you could see beyond the hills." Another voice answered, "No. Faith is such that, as you live longer, the hills become longer and higher, but you know that the road continues beyond what you can see."

The Cancer Center was patient friendly. The registrar came out to see me so I would not have to seek her out. Dr. Harvey Schick, chief radiologist and CEO of the Cancer Center, demonstrated skill, insight, and compassion. He explained the procedures. Before beginning radiation his crew had to take measurements. On my first visit, they would do a CT scan and fit me for the body cast I would wear during treatment. The cast was actually a form-fitting cradle that I would lie in for the treatments. It would permit them to aim the radiation at exactly the same spots every time. More measurements would determine the shape of the custom-made grid the technicians would place on the radiation machine to screen parts of the anatomy that they did not want to hit. They were going to target the prostate bed, because that was the most likely place for cancerous cells to be hiding and because the lymph nodes had shown no signs of malignancy.

Dr. Schick told me: "What we do is dangerous. We take special precautions to get just the right dosage at just the right place. We have the best equipment in the state right here. It allows such fine-tuning that we can get what we want and leave what we don't want."

Yet I knew that even with all the measurements, they were shooting blind. They had no proof of malignancy in the prostate bed. They were just playing the percentage game. Also, they could not leave everything that they didn't want. No matter how narrow the beam of radiation, it still must pass through part of the large intestine, burning away good cells along with the bad. That is the source of nausea, diarrhea, and those other nice things I would learn to love.

The techs calibrated the machine. They painted gun sights on my abdomen. When I got home that first day and looked in the mirror I saw, neatly painted in among the target lines, a little smiley face.

On November 15 I took the ten-minute drive to the Cancer Center for my first of thirty-five treatments. I was to go five days a week for seven weeks, which stretched into eight weeks because they let me off for Thanksgiving, Christmas, New Year's, and a blizzard. The technical staff was cheerful and considerate. In going back every day, I began to notice regular patients, many of whom looked very sick. A young mother, bald from chemo, brought her two small children with her and let them watch the proceedings on the video monitors.

The total time spent under the machine for each treatment was rarely over five minutes, but I had to block an hour and a half out of my schedule to allow time to get there from school, wait my turn, and return to school.

On an early visit, the dietician asked me to see her. She outlined the radiation-survival diet of low fiber, white bread, canned fruits, and cooked vegetables. I laughed out loud. "You are telling me to eat all the things that health gurus tell us to avoid!"

"I know. But the treatment inflames the intestines, so we don't need to have you eat high fiber foods that will further irritate the digestive track." So *bland* was the word. At first I thought, "This is no big deal." By early December the body started rebelling. The symptoms that Dr. Schick had predicted started showing themselves: diarrhea, loss of appetite, fatigue, depression. On a Saturday, after three weeks of treatment, I sat down alone to eat lunch. The sight of my sandwich made me nauseous. I broke out into sobs. "I can't eat!"

Meanwhile, I was trying to stay on top of my voice teaching at the studio and at Broad Ripple High School, getting the season going in my new church choir position and my community women's chorus, squeezing in a few storytelling engagements, and writing stories. As the treatments progressed and the fall schedule filled up, my ability to concentrate flew away. I asked Clarice to take over directing the weekly anthems with the church choir so I could focus solely on preparing and conducting our Advent cantata, the Pergolesi *Magnificat*.

Word got out that I was taking radiation. Cards, letters, and phone calls began pouring in yet again. Still, very little encouragement came from our new church, even though we had been there for six months.

Pat Mosher, a writer friend who did a lot of medical reporting, wrote me a list of questions about radiation. I was so taken by her clever and humorous slant that I wrote down answers to her questions and made up a quiz to include with our Christmas letter:

"WHAT'S HAPPENING?"

Several people have asked questions regarding the treatments I am taking. I'll answer them as best I can:

Does the treatment hurt?

No. It's just humbling.

Can they get the right target every time?

I've got gun sights painted on my abdomen (don't know where the smiley face came from, though). I'm careful not to shower around any militiamen.

Does the radiation change your behavior?
I warned my church choir that it gives me an excuse to be cranky.
Do you glow in the dark?
Not yet, but my ears get awfully hot.
Do you get X-ray vision?
I'm not saying, but the young ladies who treat me hide behind a lead shield.
Do you pick up TV signals?
The bad news is, I only get Rush Limbaugh.
Are you losing any hair?
Not anywhere you would notice.
What is it really like?
Two very attractive young women strip me and tie me down on a table. Life could be worse.

Even though I was starting to feel weak and dizzy much of the time, I could psyche myself up for special events. We got the orchestra together with the choir for the Pergolesi *Magnificat*. I feel some ownership in this music. Back in 1964 I had been the baritone soloist in the world premiere of the new edition of this work, which had been neglected for two hundred years.

[Journal, December 14, 1995] Revitalized with excellent orchestra rehearsal on Pergolesi. Can music really make us one? Two persons, who have been antagonists, created a unit of beauty. Music can be a divider. Music is capable of evil. "Music hath charms to soothe the savage beast" (or breast, whatever). Music hath power to turn one savage. Music can heal the broken. Music can destroy the whole. The creation of music can bring people together. Argument over it can destroy relationships.

The choir and orchestra responded to create a splendid performance of the first major work Clarice and I have done at Saint Andrew. Finally, the people are warming up to us.

Christmas happened, as it always does, this time with the addition of Joi's boyfriend and soon to be fiancé, Joe, Jeremy's current girlfriend, and Jon and his new bride. Missing was Mumzy, lying in the nursing home, not knowing whether it was winter or summer, day or night.

CHAPTER 13

IN FOR THE LONG HAUL

This is an entry from my journal on December 31, 1995:

Do we begin with the end in mind? Or is it end with the beginning in mind? The Romans had it right: Janus, the two-faced god looking backward and forward at the same time.

For six months my life has been controlled by cancer treatment. It is time to reclaim my life and put it to use

for family

for music

for stories

for service

The "service" part hangs me up. God, show me how.

When signs of disease would not go away, a new urgency pushed itself into an already too-crowded life: *I've got to leave some kind of legacy. Everything I have done will be diminished if I don't do something concrete.* Some people buy names for themselves on public buildings or endow arts foundations or pass on the family business. Highly unlikely in this case. After I'm gone Clarice will have to keep working just to stay afloat. My legacy is not destined to be financial. But I do have an abiding love for the enduring nature of story. I had begun a folklore study, but I had never had any of my stories published. Believing it could add a new dimension to folklore research, I threw myself into the project.

The working title became *Bullfrogs and Ezekiel: The Universal Nature of Southern Folktales*. The premise is that stories survive through generations and across cultures because they reveal something of the universal. Stories told purely for entertainment and humor often hide mythic truth. Doing the research, writing the stories, and telling the stories was fun. Submitting to a publisher was the hard part. For years I harbored a phobia about submitting manuscripts. I had earned my phobia preparing a doctoral dissertation for a sometimes hostile, always skeptical committee—on a subject about which I knew more than they did—having to explain every twitch in a five-hundred-page paper. Thereafter I had a block about submitting any writing for scrutiny.

It took twenty years, but I broke the phobia and got *Bullfrogs* into the market.

One evening early in January, I was putting up the cooking utensils and started crying. Clarice asked what was wrong. I answered, "I'm sick and tired of feeling sick and tired." She ordered me to see Dr. Lukowski immediately. I did. He started talking about antidepressant medication. I balked. I had never taken anything like that, but desperation led me to agree. He prescribed Zoloft, saying it is an antidepressant in the same class as Prozac. It regulates the production of serotonin, the hormone that affects a sense of well being. Zoloft kicks in a little faster than Prozac, and is a little milder.

On January 10 I graduated from radiation. The radiology staff all signed a "best wishes" card and gave it to me. *At last we are done with the cancer, now that they have killed off the residue in the prostate bed.*

'Twas not to be.

A month after finishing the radiation, Clarice and I went back for a follow-up with Dr. Schick. In his fatherly, compassionate way, he said: "I have some very bad news for you. Your PSA is up to 82.5."

Eighty-two point five? Before we began radiation, it had been a scant 3.0. "What do we do now?"

"First of all we'll take another PSA draw. It is most unusual for a PSA level to rise that high that quickly. We want to make sure we did not get a false reading. If it proves accurate, we have to go to another treatment. We can't radiate because we do not have a specific target. I'm confident that we got whatever residual malignancy remained in the prostate bed." Cancer cells were hiding out somewhere, but nobody knew where.

As I left Dr. Schick's office, one of the radiation technicians stopped me. "Dr. Stegall! How are you feeling?"

"I feel great, but the doc says I'm not doing too good. While you were shelling the bunkers, the bad guys escaped into the jungle. Now we are dealing with guerilla warfare."

The next PSA showed another jump, from 82.5 to 95.8, in five days' time. Dr. Schick said it was time to review options, including hormones.

I told him that I had kept, so far, my sex drive.

"I'm afraid we will cure that," he answered.

I asked, "What other side effects can I expect?"

He ticked off some of the same effects as radiation, including fatigue and depression, then added: "You'll gain weight. Your penis and testicles with shrink."

I shot back, "Lord, Harvey! If I shrink any more, I'll be an 'innie!'"

Now it was back to the urologist. Dr. Shiller went over the kinds of treatment we could use to attack the cancer in the system. Chemotherapy had not yet proven successful in fighting prostate cancer. His choice would be to starve the cancer by shutting off the supply of testosterone, which is the food of prostate cancer. He explained three basic approaches:

(1) *Using DES (diethylstilbestrol).* DES is related to the female hormone estrogen. Because DES promotes breast growth, I would have to have three doses of radiation to the breasts to prevent breast enlargement. This treatment could also cause heart problems. The good news was that it cost only about thirty dollars a month.[14]

(2) *Lupron injections.* Lupron blocks the production of testosterone in the testes. About 10 percent of the male hormones, or androgens, are produced by the adrenal glands, so he would add a daily pill to block that

source. Previously the drug of choice had been Flutamide, which one had to take three times a day. He said there was a new once-a-day drug called Casodex, which had fewer side effects than DES, but it was far more expensive: three hundred dollars a month for the shot, three hundred dollars a month for the pills.

(3) *Bilateral orchiectomy.* Castration. It would be an in-office procedure with local anesthetic. I could get it done one day, be back on the job the next. This treatment is effective.

It is also awfully permanent. We held out the hope, never mind how faint the chances, that the cancer might reverse itself, dry up, and blow away. Then we could drop the treatment, and the sex drive would re-emerge. The surgery would eliminate even that faint hope.

Dr. Shiller anticipated that within a couple of years, the cancer could find something else to feed on and start growing again, in spite of the treatment. Would the operation hold off the depression, anxiety, fatigue, increased incontinence, and diarrhea? He could not guarantee it. I would still need to take the Casodex.

He could not assure us that any of the treatments would delay the time before the cancer would become nondependent on testosterone. Nor could he assure us that the treatments would prolong life. I talked over the choices with Clarice and with our children. One son did not want to hear about it. The other said: "Dad, given those choices, it's a no-brainer. Take the pills."

Clarice said: "It's completely up to you. If insurance will cover it, do whichever feels right."

When I mentioned the treatment options to my pulmonolgist, Dr. Holmes, he shrugged and grinned. "You know, you can get prostheses to replace the testicles. They even have them for dogs!"

I choked. "Whaaa—whaat—would a neutered dog want with artificial balls?"

"I dunno. Maybe to have something to lick."

I could not wait to spring this tidbit of medical knowledge on my daughter, who worked in a veterinary clinic. She said: "Oh, yes. They come in three sizes. We have a catalog."

The next day she brought me a flyer with pictures of the fake testicles in the proper sizes for small dogs, medium-size dogs, and big dogs.

On the back were testimonials like: "My dog is so proud that he looks like other dogs." "My dog's self-confidence was very low until he got his prostheses. They have made a new dog out of him." "I don't know what my dog thinks, but I feel so much better seeing him look normal."

I decided to pass in favor of the Lupron and Casodex.

[Journal, March 8, 1996] I have just wrapped up six weeks on Zoloft for depression. I suggested to Clarice that I might ask Jack Lukowski to take me off it for a while to see what happened. She said: "I don't think so. Your behavior has been so different since you went on it, I would hate to rock the boat." I did not realize it had been so different. "Almost every day you were saying that you didn't know how you could make it. You haven't been doing that since you took the Zoloft." I reported all this to Jack when I saw him this morning. He took it as a sign to increase the dosage. His justification is that I am preparing to start Lupron injections, which is going to have some bad effects: hot flashes and, probably, mood swings. I needed a stabilizer. I said okay to increasing the dose to 100 mg. Watch out for effects of too much: nervousness and an inability to sleep.

I reported to him that Clarice had said, "If Jack asks about me, you can tell him that your wife is going crazy."

The King was not amused. Out came the Rx pad. He is also starting Clarice on 50 mg of Zoloft.

We scheduled the first Lupron injection for March 21, with Donald Shiller. I requested another PSA draw as a baseline level, because it had been a month since the last test. This time the PSA jumped another fifteen points, to 110.5. Men with metastatic inoperable cancer may not have PSAs that high.

The shot has to go deep, so the target of choice is the buttocks. The nurses are equal-opportunity administrators. They shoot the right cheek one time, the left cheek the next. After getting that first shot, the next stop was at the pharmacy to get my bottle of ten-dollar pills. That's ten dollars for *each* pill. The pharmacist scanned his computerized inventory. "How do you spell that? We don't have it. We'll order it for you." The drug was so new that they had not even stocked it. Mine was the first prescription for Casodex they had received. The pills are tiny white jobs about the size of saccharin tablets. The logo on the pill is a half-circle with an arrow. Sticks it in your face that it's going to make you "half a man."

After starting the hormones, every time we made love, I asked myself, "Is this the last time?" We made as many opportunities as possible, not knowing when it would become futile. I told Clarice repeatedly, "If I cannot reach orgasm, or lose the desire completely, I still want to provide what you need."

She would reply, "I'll let you know." Then later, "It's just not the same if we're not both in on it."

[Dream] I was going to try to play Jeremy's guitar. He said, "You'll have to restring it." I did not know how.

[Observation] If I am going to "restring" my life—make it play again—I need help. I cannot do it by myself.

[Dream, February 6, 1996] I got a partial erection. I called to Clarice, "Hey, Honey! Come look at this!"

Joi started urging us to get a smaller, one-level house. The subtext was that Dad was going to get too sick to handle stairs. We looked at a couple of houses, but said, "Not yet." Houses figured into our inner life as well. One morning Clarice awoke screaming. She sobbed hysterically for fifteen minutes. When she was calm enough, she related her dream.

[Clarice's Dream] Her house was being rearranged for her. Nothing was where it was functional. The refrigerator was in the living room, and so on. I was becoming a stranger. I was being taken away from her. She was angry at me for rearranging the house without consulting her.

If the dream house represents one's life, then Clarice's dream experience was an exact replica of the external world. Her life was being arranged in ways that she could not stop or control. She feared losing me. She was angry over the injustice of my condition's control over her life.

It would be several months before I would begin to understand the process of depression and anxiety. Antidepressants can actually create anxiety, requiring a counterbalancing antianxiety medication. Even with medication the twin demons often sucked me under.

> [Journal] Coming out of a depression is like awakening from a nightmare. The last one lasted about twenty hours—triggered about 8:00 Sunday evening, when I started gasping for air while climbing the stairs at Joe's house. That night I dreamed of being out of control. The world around me was out of focus.

> [Dream] We had bought expensive seats to a basketball game. I could not see the action. Everything was blurred. I could see movement but could not distinguish players or see whether the ball went into the basket.

I awoke with a raging headache. Had saltines and cola. Forgot to take my pills, so poured orange juice to wash them down. The pills choked me, and the juice made me nauseous. I went back upstairs and slept through my first two scheduled lessons. I managed to make it to school by around 9:00 AM. The least movement could trigger a panic attack. I would force myself to slow down and take slow, deep breaths. It worked until the next unexpected thing happened (like dropping a pencil).

I managed to teach the first lesson, then in my free hour tried to write checks for bills due and overdue. Each check precipitated gasping, shaking, even sobbing. I kept repeating, "Dear God, help me," again and again. The next lesson tugged me upward. When I had to deal with another person, I could put on the facade and act civilized.

Often—usually—when a panic attack hits, a voice in my head chastises, "Come on, man, get a grip!" Even worse, I hear Daddy grumbling at Mother: "Irma, I wish you wouldn't overdramatize so much!" That alone is enough to send one into the pits.

Amee and her husband, Sven, stood in our kitchen. I remembered the first time I was really aware of them. On one of the early fall Sundays in 1995, when Clarice and I had been at Saint Andrew for four or five months, Amee, Sven, and their two daughters marched in together and took front-row pews. During the time for sharing joys and concerns, Amee had stood up and announced: "I made a vow that when I came clean from cancer, I would do this. So, here goes!" So saying, she whipped out a kazoo and played "Jesus Loves Me."

My first impression of Amee was that she was something of a nut. Now she stood facing me in our kitchen, looking up with a face and voice full of compassion, asking me how my panic attacks manifest themselves. When I told her that they would make me stumble around, gasping and crying, sometimes screaming, she was incredulous. "I can't imagine it. You seem so calm."

I said: "Clarice can't either. It happens only when I am alone." I can comprehend why people sometimes relate that they are possessed by demons.

Meanwhile, on Monday, Clarice was depressed. She told me she was filled with self-loathing. She felt fat and lazy and unmotivated. Monday afternoon I made a special trip by her office to give her a chocolate chip cookie.

CHAPTER 14

FAMILY CRISES

O f our three children, our youngest features most in this story because he was the one at home while we were living it. When he found out that both Clarice and I were taking antidepressants, he went ballistic. "My parents! Taking mind-altering drugs! After all you have said about coke and pot, now you are becoming junkies!" A few weeks later he had an appointment to see Dr. Lukowski. Our son came back with a good report on his own health, but then exploded. "You betrayed me! You lied to me!"

"What are you talking about?"

"You didn't tell me you were sick!"

I thought, *What on earth has Jack told him?* But I answered: "We have informed you of every step in the treatment. We clued you in on the surgery, the radiation, and the hormone treatments."

"But you didn't tell me that you were dying!"

Jack had told our son that his father was "not a well man." He had described to him the possibilities of where the cancer could go and what the prognosis would be if it went to the bones.

"It goes into bone cancer. You can't cure bone cancer!" Our macho eighteen-year-old with the hair down to his waist, who wore combat boots and leather jackets—our baby child—was terrified.

No honest parent will claim that raising children is easy. I thank God again and again for the blessings we have in our children. It is the struggle itself that creates the blessing. Our older son had survived burning anger over being abandoned in Korea. He had overcome his hatred of "high school prison" to flourish in college and establish a budding accounting career. Our daughter's Korean heritage never seemed to concern her. She tried different college majors, but her dream was of becoming a veterinarian.

This younger son, with his phenomenal musical gifts, athletic ability, and a mind that always asked the unexpected questions, knew he was not in sync with the system. On a sunny spring day when he was in eighth grade, he and I had gone to play tennis after school. While we were looking for a court, he told me that his English teacher had taken him out in the hall and demanded to know why he had not done the assignment for the day. My son's answer: "Because I am a lateral thinker and you are a linear thinker, and I think your way is stupid."

Once when a counselor asked him what he liked doing, he answered, "Being with my friends and playing my guitar."

He finally made it to his senior year. He developed some good friendships. Many weekend nights he and his friends would sit around his fire pit in the backyard, playing guitars and singing until the early hours of the morning.

We still were in constant stress as to whether he would graduate. One more failing grade and he wouldn't.

One night I went to bed early. My son was down in the den watching television. I had just settled into my first good snooze. A distinct inner voice jolted me awake: *Go down and see your son.* The bed was comfortable. The thermostat was turned down, and the house was cooling off for the night. I snuggled deeper under the comforter and dozed off.

Again I felt those words: *Go down and see your son.*

The voice had a quiet urgency. I remembered the story of Samuel.[15] *That voice is going to keep calling until I pay attention. I may as well get it over with. No point waiting for the third call.*

Grumbling, I dragged myself out from under my warm comforter, groped around for my slippers, and stumbled to the closet to get my robe.

I was still foggy as I felt my way down two flights to the den. The bright TV screen flickered on my son's forlorn face. The program was

Deep Space Nine, a *Star Trek* spin-off. I liked this show, though I rarely saw it. I told my son that I had not been able to sleep, so I would just sit with him for a while. He made no acknowledgment.

Having no clue what to say, but knowing that I had to be there at that moment, I turned my attention to the TV show.

One of the space crew had a son who was studying to enter the space academy. The son passed all the tests. Then he said to his dad: "I don't want it. I don't want the academy. I didn't tell you earlier because I was afraid you would be angry."

The father put his hand on the boy's shoulder. "All I want is for you to find what you really love, and do it with all your heart."

I knew I had my message. Neither my son nor I said anything until the commercial break. Then I turned to him and touched my hand to his knee. "That's all I want for you: to find what you really love, and do it with all your heart."

"Thanks."

The program returned. He left to go to bed. I stayed and watched the end.

Friday, May 31, 1996, was my son's last day of high school. He went to school that day not knowing whether he would graduate. Midmorning my phone rang. It was Clarice. Her voice was on a trampoline. "Honey! He made it!" His counselor had just called Clarice at work to tell her. I was already planning to take him to lunch at his favorite lunch-treat restaurant, Red Lobster, to celebrate the end of school. When he got in the car, I said, "Well, congratulations, Graduate!"

He shrugged. "I guess."

He did not know! I was the one to give him the good news! I heard myself speaking. I was restrained, almost matter-of-fact. I sounded like my daddy! *Oh, my God! Why can I not show him how excited I am?*

That evening my son had some friends over to celebrate the end of school. They were sitting around his fire pit enjoying a nice bonfire when Clarice got home. She called him up to the deck. They embraced. They both cried. I was thrilled, but felt left out.

I was now determined that my son would know that his dad really cared. We made a big hoopla about graduation. When his class, all 780-plus, marched into Market Square Arena, our son was not to be missed. He was the guy with golden tresses flowing freely across his shoulders and down below his shoulder blades. He was the one flashing us his gazillion-dollar grin as he returned to his seat with his diploma.

After it was all official, diploma in hand and all, I ventured to him: "I am so proud of your sticking with school. My great fear was that you would give up and drop out."

"Dad, I would never do that."

Payoffs come late, in surprise packages. Weeks later our son told us about one of his friends from school. He had been living with his grandmother, who had told him that he was on his own after high school. Now our son's friend had nowhere to go. "He doesn't have a good family like I have," he told us matter-of-factly.

CHAPTER 15

DUEL BETWEEN MIND AND SPIRIT

Meanwhile, the professional life kept blowing its whistles at us. We were also spending many hours on the upcoming 1996 ADM church music workshop in Tulsa, Oklahoma. "We" includes Clarice, because I, in an act of blatant nepotism, had appointed her worship chairperson. Preparations for the workshop seeped into every part of my consciousness and my unconscious.

> [Dream] The ADM workshop was in session. I was a mess. I could not read a sentence straight. I was trying to make announcements. I kept stumbling. I apologized to Danny (the president). I knew he would never ask me to do anything again.

Coming to grips with the disease meant making some fundamental commitments with the rest of my life. We do not live in a vacuum. Illness is not a separate compartment. Intricate relationships opened up for me on a spring walk in the park:

> [Journal] A picnic table down on the riverbank.
> A dead tree stands in the water.
> What good does a dead tree do?
> A bird sings in the bare branches.
> The tree provides a resting place for the bird.
> It provides food for woodpeckers.

Another maple tree lies fallen into the water,
broken off from its roots and rotting.
But—one live branch grows up from the side of the trunk.
New leaves sprout from the branch.
The bottom side of the trunk is under the water.
New roots must have put down in the water.
There in Broad Ripple Park,
by the side of the White River,
I do not have to stretch far
to ignore the surrounding city.
I sit on a picnic table and talk to God.
Out loud.

God, I know you can heal me of cancer and of (after three-and-a-half years, I still do not have a proper label. To control it I must be able to *name* it—so "lung crud" it shall be) lung crud. May I do my part—
Proper diet
Proper exercise
Humor
Thankfulness
Service? Service? Did I hear you say, "Service?"

Go to Africa? How about what I'm already doing—affirming young lives by teaching them a skill that will tap into the core being; opening up vistas of imagination and remembrance as people hear, and share, stories; bringing understanding to a reading audience through my folk-lore study?

Or should I go out and raise ten thousand dollars for the March of Dimes, like that priest did from his hospital room?

"Show love to all?" That's easy: Clarice, our children, their wife/fiancé/girlfriend, Mumzy. Can I draw the line at K? I don't have to like someone to love them, right? Okay—I'll accept K. Love could follow. Then maybe, just maybe, I could learn to like him.

"Pray for people other than myself?" Okay. But I need to be specific. "All our missionaries in foreign fields" doesn't cut it. I'll begin with D. May she have a safe pregnancy and deliver a healthy child(ren). Then R. and H. May they find the proper solution to their childlessness. Oh, yes—the family—make sure they are well taken care of. That is the most emotional concern I have about them.

"Accept the lack of a sex drive as a blessing?" I know, I know. I can focus more on my job without being distracted by lust. But I enjoy lust! Besides, now I am not doing what my *wife* needs! We have a strange role reversal here.

"Accept morning sickness, hot flashes, PMS?"

All this just to put my life in your hands?

May I do what I must.

May I let go of what I must.

The single greatest parable of faith I have ever seen was Indiana Jones in the film *Indiana Jones and the Last Crusade*, stepping out into what appeared to be a chasm, only to find it to be a camouflaged bridge.

"You don't know until you try." Is that what you are telling me?

The school year ended. On the first day of summer break, I took a long walk along Fall Creek. I wanted to spend the day on my folklore research, so I tried to think about it as I walked. "Sody Salaraytus"[16] is a humorous/fantastic Southern tale about a squirrel who rescues an entire family: "the little woman, the little man, the little girl, the little boy, him and his sody salaraytus," from the belly of a bear.

I could not bring any coherent thought to the surface.

I observed the water, the currents, debris, joining branches of the creek, and rapids. Nearing the rapids the water becomes faster, more turbulent, and then the surface smoothes out, looking like molded glass. Then comes the bubbling and rush across the rocks.

No research idea came.

I observed trees on the bank whose roots were gradually being exposed. No matter how big or tenacious the tree, the water will eventually win.

No new idea emerged.

Near the end of the walk, I gave up. *Sometimes, they say, if you let your mind go blank, ideas will emerge.* The mind, however, would not go blank. It just wandered from the mud in the path to the maintenance men spraying the trees.

Reward.

As I neared the car, the idea leapt out. *Reward.* What reward does the hero receive in "Sody Salaraytus"? It fell into place. Good must fight evil. Good must win. Good must be rewarded. The heroic little squirrel in this humorous folktale gets the proper reward: "three whole sody-biscuits." Bread, the staff of life. The reward is strength to keep living! *Is that what one can expect for prevailing over death? No gold? No fame? Just—the strength to keep living? Isn't that enough? I think for me, right now, it is sufficient. To live fully, to rejoice in life in the face of loss.*

At that moment my loss was specific. The nerves of sexual arousal would no longer respond. I had hoped that even if the drive was gone, the nerves could be stimulated to excitement. That was no longer to be.

[Dream, June 7, 1996] A broken mirror and a broken glass pedestal. The boy who broke the pedestal apologized, but then proceeded to continue smashing it. He said it was trash anyway.

[Observation] Does the broken pedestal relate to castration? Is the boy my impulsive child? Why does he continue breaking the glass?

It had been exactly a year since Dr. Shiller had called to tell me they had found a "moderately aggressive malignancy."

Dear God, I accept whatever is best for me and for my family. I don't know the answers. I know you can cure. There is already healing. Clarice and I have never been so close as we are now. I enjoy life more than I ever have. By being honest about the disease that won't go away, maybe I'm helping someone else. When one talks of receiving a miraculous cure, they can't say honestly, "This, too, will happen to you."

"Who'll be a witness for my Lord?" The one who endures is a better witness than one who is cured! But I don't want disease. I don't want to be a martyr. I don't want anyone feeling sorry for me! Yuck!

Of all the dangers I have so far encountered, I fear Demon Martyrdom the most. A voice calls from somewhere in the unconscious: "Good people suffer. You suffer because you are good. People look at you and say, 'O how brave!'" When I hear that voice, I shudder. I know that voice. It is Mother. She, as we say in the family, enjoyed poor health. She did have diabetes, leukemia, phlebitis, angina, high blood pressure, and whatever else was in vogue. She dragged herself through at least thirty years with enough wrong with her to kill a healthy person. When she died, the friends gathered for the litany of "how brave Miz Stegall was."

When my brother, Joel, and I were boys, friends of Mother and Daddy liked to ruffle our hair and exclaim, "Joel is just like his daddy, and Carroll is just like his mother."

I would bite my lip and look over at Joel to see him clamping his jaw and staring at the ground. Those words have haunted me to the present day. When some well-meaning person praises me for "handling the disease so well," part of me tries to accept it graciously, but another part screams, *Please don't try to make me a martyr!*

CHAPTER 16

A LOSE/LOSE GAME

It came time to get the first PSA draw since beginning the hormone treatment. Dr. Shiller had wanted to give it three months. I went into this one with some dread. *It's a lose/lose game. If the reading is still up, it says the hormone treatment is not working, so we may as well discontinue it. If the reading is down, it says the hormone treatment is working, so why not go ahead and snip those balls off and be done with it?*

Clarice went with me to this appointment. Dr. Shiller strode in, brisk as ever. He was not pleased with the news he had to give. The PSA was down from 110 to 67. That was not good enough. After three months he had expected it to be below 10.

"So you suspect that it has hit bottom and is back on the rise?"

"That's what I suspect." He reminded me that 15 percent of men with prostate cancer have a strain that is resistant to hormone therapy. "We will retake the PSA in a month. If it is lower, we will keep on the hormones. If it is higher, we will send you to an oncologist for third-line therapies." At that point they would also do another bone scan to check for "hot spots." "Should symptoms appear, if there is anything you have always wanted to do but have never done, I urge you to do it as soon as possible." Once the cancer spreads to the bones, the survival expectancy is two to five years.

Gomella and Fried, in *Recovering from Prostate Cancer*, raise another complication:

The hormone therapy will not affect those cancerous cells—thought to include as many as 10 to 20 percent—that are not hormone dependent or hormone sensitive. These cells, left to themselves, would go on reproducing. In fact, because they no longer face competition from the testosterone-dependent cancerous cells, the non-hormone-dependent cells may expand their domain, reproducing geometrically to grow into the space once occupied by the hormone-dependent sisters."[17]

I said, "Donald, I am not afraid of dying. I never have been. I am afraid of pain. I am afraid of becoming dependent. I am afraid of leaving my family in bad straits."

A few days later our older son Jon, the CPA, came for a four-day visit. I told Jon about the latest PSA and the possible future scenario. His response was to question the statistical studies. He said: "I guess it's the accountant in me. I have to question and poke holes until I'm satisfied the data is sound."

Jon's questions confronted fundamental issues. It is true that prostate cancer grows slowly. It is true that natural causes often take lives before the prostate cancer gets to the life-threatening stage. It is true that the PSA, the best early-warning signal we currently have, is an inexact marker. It is also true that I am in the statistical minority: PSA dropped, then rose again after surgery, continued rising after radiation, then stayed high after three months of hormone therapy.

[Dream, June 16, 1996] A man was imprisoned in a dungeon. The jailer took everything he had, but missed a jeweled cross the man wore around his neck. I saw the cross fall out of his shirt collar and dangle outside the bars, glinting in a thin stream of sunlight. It was a dark Celtic cross inset with deep purple stones. The prisoner managed to pull the cross back into his shirt without the jailer seeing him. I had an ominous feeling that the jailer would eventually find the cross and steal it, too.

[Observation] Can the cross symbolize faith and life? As Scrooge said, "Is this a portent of what must be, or only what might be?" I *have* a new day. It is even Father's Day. I will live each day as if it were the first discovery of love!

Father's Day dinner, 1996. Jon, Joi, and her boyfriend, Joe, Jeremy,[18] and his girlfriend, Joe's dad (his mom was visiting friends in California), Clarice and I all had dinner at our house. It was on that same Father's Day that Dumb Old Dad couldn't catch on to the message Joi kept flashing to me. When Joe served champagne, Joi held the glasses in a peculiar manner, her fingers on top instead of around the stem, so Joe had to pour the champagne between her fingers. I thought it looked amusing, so I tried it. When he filled my glass, I held my fingers over the top like Joi had done. Everyone was holding their sides laughing. Jeremy's face ran with tears of laughter. *This is a peculiar practice, but is it that funny?*

Finally Jeremy could not stand it anymore. "Dad! Look at her finger!" The laughter reached near hysteria. Then I saw. Joi had been flashing her diamond ring at me for two days, but I had been looking at where she was pointing, not at her hand! Jeremy sputtered, "I'll remember this for the rest of my life!"

After dinner I took Jeremy aside and told him about the latest medical word. In his usual terse way, he replied, "Thank you for letting me know." That evening he and Clarice would still be ribbing me about my slowness in recognizing Joi's grand news. Jeremy said, "You gave me a good laugh, and I thank you for it."

In the afternoon Jon, Joi, and Joe all joined me to watch the Chicago Bulls win their fourth NBA championship. After the Bulls defeated the Sonics, Michael Jordan fell prostrate on the floor, sobbing. A reporter asked him how he felt. His answer, choked with sobs, was that his wife and children are the most important thing in the world to him, and that this, his fourth NBA championship, was the sweetest because he dedicated it to his father (murdered two years before), and they won it on Father's Day.

I thought, *This man has his priorities right.*

On that Father's Day, I witnessed Michael Jordan's commitment to his family, a commitment that overrode his unprecedented athletic feat. That same day I felt the love and laughter of rich family ties that overrode health anxieties. We are not playing lose/lose unless the physical dimension is the only dimension that matters. We win, not by denying or fighting the physical choices, but by rising to another dimension.

Clarice and I decided to take Dr. Shiller's prompting literally, and do things we had put off. For Memorial Day weekend, we drove down into Kentucky to spend two days at Shaker Village. There we slowed down. We walked. We talked. We snuggled against the brisk spring breeze. We witnessed the dying arts of quilting, furniture building, and broom making. We attended a re-enactment of a Shaker meeting, experiencing the simple songs and dances that grew spontaneously out of a people who believed and practiced, "Hands to work; hearts to God."

It was from the Shakers that the song "Simple Gifts" arose. Aaron Copland used it in his ballet *Appalachian Spring*, as well as in *Old American Songs*, which he wrote for the renowned baritone William Warfield.

Now, hearing "Simple Gifts" stripped of orchestral color and sung unaccompanied by a lovely, untrained voice, pointed me to where I needed to go.

'Tis the gift to be simple, 'tis the gift to be free,
'Tis the gift to come down where we ought to be.
And when we find ourselves in the place just right,
'Twill be in the valley of love and delight.
When true simplicity is gained,
To bow and to bend we shan't be ashamed.
To turn, turn will be our delight,
'Till by turning, turning, we come round right.[19]

The song makes complete sense when it becomes a dance. It is full of images of gentle movement: bowing, bending, turning.

It is no "Onward, Christian soldiers, marching as to war,"[20] or even a "Jacob's Ladder,"[21] where we climb "higher, higher," until we reach our heavenly goal. The righteous life is not found by going out into the battlefield. The righteous life is not found in determining a goal and stubbornly striving toward it. The righteous life finds you where you are as you work, pray, sing, and dance. Little wonder that "Simple Gifts" became the defining song of the Shaker movement. Little wonder that "Hands to work; hearts to God" became their mission statement.

As tourist places go, there is "nothing to do" in Shaker Village. Even so, we did not want to leave. But we had jobs to get back to, a mortgage to pay, and a family to care for.

CHAPTER 17

SEEKING A SPIRITUAL MENTOR

I had not been active in my urology group's support group. It met on an evening when I had a heavy teaching load. The group was too large to accommodate the personal sharing I needed. In June 1996, after three months on the new hormone treatment, the PSA remained high. Urinary leakage increased. Morning sickness continued to nag. Even with all those considerations, it took Donald Shiller's wake-up call—"Do everything you've always wanted to do"—to frighten me into attending the June meeting. As we gathered in the meeting room, Clarice and I looked around. Nearly all the men there were ten to twenty years older than I was. During the discussion, several of them expressed concerns about their rising PSAs, in the range of 6.0 to 10.0. I whispered to Clarice: "I'm the champ! I'm the Michael Jordan of this gathering! Not one has a PSA that can touch my high of 110.5."

Living with a mysterious autoimmunity as well as cancer further complicated the issues. Dr. Shiller had observed that my depression was the most intense he had ever seen. Those new twists prodded me to seek counseling. Clarice did not deserve to be the dumpee all the time. My counselor of choice was Cyndi Alte. She is not only a former hospice nurse and a current pastor, but also a valued and trusted friend.

In our first session, she confronted my sense of detachment and lack of obvious anger. *I'm supposed to be angry? Am I just in denial?*

Observing that I may need some off-hours help, she volunteered to give me all her phone numbers, so I could get in touch with her anytime or anyplace. Then she gave a sheepish grin. "I've got to let you in on one of my little secrets. I don't have anything to hook my beeper to, so I have it hooked on my slip. Please excuse me while I retrieve it." As she spoke she hiked up her skirt to get to her beeper.

How am I supposed to contemplate my anger if I can't stop laughing? Am I weird, or what?

I told her, "I am trying to learn how to approach prayer." For quite a long time in my adult life, I did not think of prayer as anything other than giving oneself a pep talk or a dressing down. When I did pray, I felt a visceral tension between petition and acceptance.

Then, the night before I was to meet with Cyndi, I had remembered Jesus' prayer in the Garden of Gethsemane: "Father, if you are willing, remove this cup from me; yet, not my will but yours be done."[22] Jesus himself hit both sides of petition and acceptance! I shared this observation with Cyndi.

She pressed the issue further. She has seen people die who should not. She has seen people live who were not expected to. She said: "What happens between 'Let this cup pass from me' and 'Your will be done'? I don't think it is simply a semicolon. Something else happens."

Listening. That's it. Listening. Waiting. There is even more. If prayer is an ongoing conversation and not confined to a moment of clasped hands and closed eyes, action also enters in. I had never before tried to tie procedure and goals to prayer. A whole new world beckoned.

I told Cyndi that Clarice and I had each independently calculated that if my PSA came down four points a day between the last blood test and the next one in October, it would be at zero.

Cyndi and I devised what she called the four-point prayer. We would pray that the PSA would come down four points each day. But the four points were more fundamental than the specific request. We vowed to pray:
- *Believing* that God can grant a desired result,
- *Specifically* for that result,
- *Waiting*, listening, doing everything in our power to clear the path for healing,
- *Accepting* whatever outcome God grants.

Cyndi instructed me to meditate on Genesis 3:21: "The Lord God made garments of skin for Adam and his wife and clothed them."

I asked, "What does this obscure verse have to do with me?" After stewing over it awhile, the truth hit. "Of course! They had to leave Paradise and go out into a hostile, unknown world, but God prepared them and protected them."

By the end of our session, I was still puzzled by her confrontation of my detachment. I did not feel that I was detached.

Then a story from my deep past leapt to the front of consciousness. Not knowing quite why, I felt the need to relate to Cyndi an event that had happened more than thirty years before.

When I was in high school back in St. Pauls, North Carolina, Daddy was fired from his pastorate. That was in 1957. I was not quite sixteen. He took whatever work he could, including measuring croplands and cleaning out tobacco barns. During that time he went for counseling with the "First Baptist" pastor, Dr. D. Swan Hayworth.

Several years later, in 1963, when I was applying to graduate schools, one of my options was music study in seminary. Dr. Hayworth wrote a letter in support of my application for a scholarship to the Southern Baptist Theological Seminary in Louisville, Kentucky. I also applied for scholarships at the Manhattan School of Music in New York, then decided I would go wherever I got the best offer.

The seminary did not award me a scholarship. The conservatory did, so it was off to New York to work on a master of music degree in vocal performance. Being a good Baptist, one of the first things I did when I got to New York was to seek out the Manhattan Baptist Church. My first Sunday there, the guest minister was none other than Dr. Hayworth.

In his sermon he related the story of a pastor who had come to him for counseling. Dr. Hayworth told us that in their early sessions, this pastor had remained calm in revealing the difficulties he was experiencing. Finally, after several weeks, he had cried out:

"My God! Why is this happening to me?"

Chills went up my back. Dr. Hayworth was talking about my daddy! I could hardly contain myself when I went up to reintroduce myself to Dr. Hayworth after church. He had not seen me there, so greeted me with surprise. "Well, Stegall! So you are going to the conservatory instead of seminary. I can't understand why the seminary did not give you that scholarship. I don't see how anyone could have been better qualified."

I thanked him for his gracious endorsement, then went straight to the burning question. "Dr. Hayworth, was that Daddy you were talking about?" His jovial face turned somber. He looked down at the floor. He played with his lower lip. Then he looked up, facing me squarely. "Well, your father did have some difficult times that he talked with me about."

No need to press him further. I knew that this chance meeting had provided a portrait of Daddy I had never known.

The evening after the first session with Cyndi, I prepared a letter to her:

Dear Cyndi: You raised the question of anger. There is something in there shouting, "No fair!" The men I know personally who have had prostate surgery are all at least ten years older than I am, and all have tested out clear. That's the way it is supposed to go. This form of cancer does not, as yet, demonstrate any particular cause and effect, such as one sees in lung cancer. It appears to be completely democratic, or completely capricious, depending on how you see those things.

You prayed on this order: "Be with Carroll as he faces his death." I realize I must do that before I can fully live. I have told Clarice a few times that I don't know whether I am in denial or just numb, but when we have gotten one piece of bad news or another, it has been almost as if the doctor were talking about someone else.

I did not think of the intimate connection of the story I told you about my father and Dr. Hayworth until I was telling it to you. Part of its impact was in realizing that I was, in relating that anecdote, vicariously screaming out to you, "My God! Why is this happening to me?"

I want my beloved children to know me as I really am. I want to be able to reveal it myself, without having to wait for someone else to tell me, as Dr. Hayworth did for me.

I relish the affection Joi has been lavishing on me. I hope it is mainly due to her being so happy that she and Joe are engaged. The poignant part is my sensing that she is also signaling a fear of losing me.

I am entering a new world. The liberal skeptic has always kept the rope of his hot-air balloon tied to a tree. He has never really cut that rope and let the balloon fly. May he have the faith to cut it loose! Carroll

Since 1981 I have kept, with varying degrees of regularity, a journal of thoughts, events, and dreams. Dreams often reveal insights into specific events. At the second session with Cyndi, we talked about how we can learn from dreams. It triggered another letter.

Dear Cyndi: You asked about my dreams. This is from last night. The dream is based on a real circumstance. My last year (1964–65) at the Manhattan School of Music, which at that time was in Spanish Harlem on East 106th Street in New York, I lived alone in an apartment in a building owned by the school. The building, a five-level storefront walk-up, was right around the corner from the school on Second Avenue. It was a slum area. The apartments were managed by the school bursar, Stanley Bednar. Here is the dream:

I was back in school. Mr. Bednar announced that our building was going to be renovated. The day arrived when I would move from my old apartment into a newly renovated space.

I had several roommates, male and female. When we entered the new room, we gasped. It was fully carpeted with plush gray carpet. It was furnished with antiques. In the center of the room was a six-foot Steinway grand piano. (When I told this part to Clarice, she retorted, "In your sweet dreams!") *Over in the right corner was what looked like a harpsichord. A pot of water was boiling on the stove, brewing fresh tea. I thought, "That's a nice gesture of welcome, but that tea is going to be too strong."*

Examining the room, I walked over to the "harpsichord" and lifted the lid. It really was Clarice's baby high chair. (We still have that chair. She used it, her brother used it, and so did Joi and Jeremy.[23])

I looked around the luxurious setting and observed, "He did not raise the rent on us. I have gone from squalor to luxury in one day, and it didn't cost a cent!"

In the far left corner was a studio-type kitchen. I saw that the gas stove was on, but now nothing was cooking. I said, "That can be dangerous," and reached to turn off the burner. Another burner came on. Every time I turned

one off, another came on. In addition, the number of burners multiplied, until the stove had maybe a dozen burners.

In thinking about the "new digs," Jesus's words came immediately to mind: "In my Father's house there are many dwelling places."[24]

The antique furnishings in a new place tie past with present and future.

The piano. It was our six-foot Steinway, our most prized earthly possession. It was proper for that piece to be in the center of the room. Music is the center of our lives.

The high chair. I don't know why it started out as a harpsichord, but the chair is one of our physical generational connections. Life continues, regardless of what happens to any individual.

The stove. There's something sinister about that stove. It was positioned wrong. It was out of place, pulled away from the wall and angled back toward the cabinet where it could not be reached for cooking. It kept sprouting, not only new flames but also new burners. I knew, in my dream, that the flame that should serve me as a means of cooking, could, instead, cook me and the dwelling.

The misplaced, reproducing stove fits my understanding of what happens with cancer—cells that are designed to be beneficial get out of place and go into uncontrolled growth. One can kill it off in one spot, only to have it crop up somewhere else, or again at the same place.

The multiple roommates whose names I do not now know. There is much about my own life that I do not yet know. But wherever I go, all these unconscious companions, male and female, are there, too.

The tea my unseen host was brewing was not done my way. I felt resentment that I wasn't able to brew it the way I wanted it. I was not in control.

This was a new apartment, not a house: I don't own it. This "apartment," this body, is entrusted to me. God is preparing an improved body for me. Is this a signal for a return to health, or is it telling me of a "new body" in resurrection? Or was the whole thing caused by too much pizza?

Love, Carroll

CHAPTER 18

ON THE MOVE

J uly 1996. ADM Church music workshop time with a difference. This year I was in charge. I had worked for two years
toward this one week. Clarice had planned the daily chapel
services. I had lined up clinicians and teachers and set up the schedule.
All the planning council members had assigned duties. Two hundred and
fifty musicians were gathering for a week of learning, inspiration, fellowship, and fun. The heat was so intense in Tulsa that, as people gathered to
register, one of our enterprising women stood at the door of the residence
hall with a spritzer bottle and sprayed everyone with water as they
entered.

I had now been on the hormone treatments for four months. The
predicted side effects were daily companions. As the entire crowd gathered for our opening reception on Saturday evening, I decided to handle
the repeated questions of "Well, how *are* you?" all at one time. When I
took the microphone to welcome people and to introduce our guest clinicians (faculty), I said:

"Those of you who were here last year observed, on occasion, that I
looked a little gray." Good-natured chuckles rippled around the room. "Since
then I have had radiation and now have started on hormone treatments. So
I am getting accustomed to this wonderful new world of morning sickness,
mood changes, and—hot flashes." The room erupted in laughter. That's what
I wanted. To tell the truth and put people at ease at the same time.

Beth, one of my cronies who did not come until the next day, got a report on my announcement of the previous evening. When I first saw her, she hugged me and exclaimed, "So, you'll have PMS just like the rest of us!"

"That's right, sister!"

Clarice and I continued to take Dr. Shiller's advice to do things we had put off. In 1971 and 1973, when we were graduate students with money and no children, we had gone to the Stratford Festival in Stratford, Ontario, tent-camping at the town fairgrounds. Now it was time to make that long-awaited return trip. But no tent this time. We stayed at a bed and breakfast.

We saw five plays in four days, including Shakespeare's *King Lear*. I read the script ahead of time. I had never seen *King Lear*. I almost dreaded it—long, dark, brooding, tragic. With my increasing bouts with depression, would it be too much? But nothing prepared me for the dazzling production. Nothing prepared me for the mesmerizing humanity of Lear as played by William Hutt. Nothing prepared me for the lightning flashes of humor that showed us the whole picture, not just the shadows.

I experienced what the Greek tragedies set out to accomplish. I experienced horror and pity, out of which came cleansing. How could I, as a father, not identify with the selfish father who could not bear to share his daughter's love with another man? How could I, as a fair-minded human, not identify with Cordelia, the daughter who honestly confesses her true love to her father?

Tears and laughter are twins.

At our hosts' suggestion, Clarice and I enjoyed our twenty-eighth anniversary dinner in a quiet little restaurant that was set up like a home. We dined in upholstered wingback chairs at a dining table next to a fireplace. A bookcase filled with classics stood by my chair. It was quite different from some of our earlier anniversary meals, cooked over Sterno in front of our tent.

Just as we had done twenty-three years earlier, we took a paddleboat out on the Avon River. Only this time we did not have a beagle along. We walked along the river walk where we had once tried to teach our beagle to swim, a beagle who hated the water. This time the main entertainment was a pair of swans engaging in a domestic quarrel. For all their beauty, swans are not gentle animals. We watched part of a lawn bowling tournament. We drove to a secluded, fenced lake where the legendary single pair of black swans lived in haughty solitude. For the past three years, their eggs had been destroyed, vandalized by human hands. Because swans lay only two eggs a year, these magnificent creatures were now under police protection.

By now our anniversary was short on sex. That aspect of our life was in deep hibernation. Clarice's understanding and acceptance made the loss bearable. But the anniversary was long on affection, nostalgia, and planning for the future.

Clarice had never traveled abroad. I had done so only once. Our wake-up call set us in motion planning to fulfill other dreams. Some time later we discovered that a friend was putting together a tour to attend the Oberammergau Passion Play in 2000. The little German village of Oberammergau, in the Bavarian Alps, has staged all-day presentations of the Passion every ten years since 1634, when it was spared from the Black Plague. We decided to sign on for this millennial production.

CHAPTER 19

THE BULLS IN THE CASTLE

Dream, July 27, 1996, ca. 2:30 PM] In this dream I face death. The dream seems to connect at almost every point with the cancer. In the dream I face the fear that I had denied while I was awake. It is a different fear from anything I had experienced before. Having been told, "You will die tonight," I prepare for it. Then comes the unsettling thought: "What if I don't die? If I keep living, after coming to the brink, life will never be the same." The dream structures itself in the form of a play, with a prologue, three acts, two entr'actes, and an epilogue. I present it here, with no elaboration, the way I remember it.

Prologue

Part A

The doctor told me I would die before morning. I knew it would happen eventually. But so soon? I had not even felt sick. I wanted something to remind me of Mother. So they decorated a bathroom with some of her pictures.

I started repeating, again and again: "O God, I'm scared."

Then—"What if I wake up? What if I don't die? After preparing myself and my family for death? If it doesn't happen, life will be very different from what it was." That prospect was almost as unsettling as the other.

Part B

Our new Honda got a dent on the fender in front of the right rear wheel. I wanted to get it fixed so I could sell it. I needed to drive the car down to the body shop. It kept slipping off the road, then going down blind hallways (not alleys; it was inside a building).

Act 1

A young performance artist staged a horseback bullfight. The exhibition took place in the brick-paved enclosed courtyard of a Spanish castle. I stood with other spectators inside the building, protected by walls. We looked out through windows. The performance artist was dressed like a toreador. He had the heroic appearance of a Tristan-like young warrior. His father was the director of the performance. Occasionally the bulls broke out of the courtyard into the villa, but they did not come near me.

Entr'acte

Another father-son team put on a performance in an auditorium. They had rigged up a waterslide on the stage. The father went first, plunging headfirst down the slide and off the stage. The audience gasped. We thought he was going to bash his head on the floor in front of the stage. Instead, he bounced safely on a mattress. We laughed in relief.

Act 2

Now it was winter. An arts event was going to restage the equestrian bullfight, but now it was no longer just a bullfight. It was a civil war that spread throughout the castle. The warriors, wearing toreador uniforms, used horses, lances, and bulls in the fight. The Young Warrior's father was no longer in charge. Rather, a woman like the Queen of Hearts was the commander. The battle raged on the courtyard level of the castle. I told my friends that they should be safe if they stayed on the top floor and looked out over the balconies.

Entr'acte

Another staging of the waterslide trick. This time the son was the performer. We expected him to slide off the stage and bounce on the mattress in the same manner as had his father. But he came up with a trick or two of his own. He slid headfirst off the stage, hit another water chute, and propelled himself up the side aisle (stage right), out the door, and out of sight. Again, surprised laughter and applause from us in the audience.

Act 3

No sooner had I told my friends that we would be safe on the balconies than the bulls and warriors came charging up the stairs to the upper levels. They had not gotten to our level yet, but I now knew we were in mortal danger. The warriors were fighting among themselves. The young warrior led one army. They were all dressed alike, so I did not know how they knew whom to attack. As they fought among themselves, the bulls ran free, rampaging throughout the castle.

I was now on the top level of the castle. The warriors invaded the roof, which was flat, like a balcony. Some of the warriors tried to leave the battle. On the balcony roof, over to the side near the edge, was a small cupola with a low, A-frame red tile roof. I saw warriors on the left side of the cupola starting to push on the roof, attempting to push it off the cupola. If they succeeded it would crash into the courtyard below. I thought the Young Warrior was with the defecting warriors, hanging on the other side of the roof. I ran around to try to save him. Instead, he became captain of the group that was pushing the roof off.

When I got around to the other (right) side, I saw, hanging from the edge, not warriors, but five clown puppets. I could not fight off the warriors on the other side who were pushing on the roof. I grabbed hold of the feet of the first puppet. The puppets' legs were like the woven crepe paper legs of paper clown dolls. The clown puppet outfits were, I knew, costumes. I pulled off the costume legs of the first puppet. It was a young child, frightened, hanging on because it did not know anything else to do. I then pulled the costume legs off the next puppet. This one, also, ceased to act like a puppet, and became a frightened child.

The puppet master appeared and started to fight me off. I grabbed his legs and pulled off his costume. He then realized that he had been as much a slave as the children had been. He had been a puppet controlling puppets to do what his master had wanted. He became my ally, assisting in pulling the costumes off the remaining children.

Now they were all children, no longer puppets. Yet they were not safe. They were clinging desperately to the edge of the roof as it was pushed closer and closer to the edge. I told them to jump. They couldn't. "I'll fall into the courtyard and be killed," one pleaded.

"No! There's a ledge here. I'm standing on it. Just let go and drop onto the ledge."

But they could not let go. The puppet master and I pulled on their legs, one child at a time, to stretch them down to where they could feel the concrete ledge under their toes. Each, in turn, stood safely on the ledge. Just as the last one jumped down, the roof sailed over our heads and crashed into the courtyard far below.

Epilogue

I went to a concert. A sixtyish man, square of build, with a crewcut, was there. I recognized him as the one who had bought my car. Said he: "You never owned that car. There was a form you didn't sign. So it wasn't legal for you to sign it to me." I laughed. I thought it was amusing.

This dream is one of the most complex, and most thoroughly structured, dreams I have ever experienced. It is certainly rare to have an introduction, then a-b-a-b-a with a coda—a perfect musical rondo form!

The dream itself provoked many questions, but thinking about it keeps raising more. I sensed, even while the dream was progressing, that something significant was happening. What is going on here? Let's first have a go at the characters and places.

The bulls. At first controlled, even choreographed, they rampage in the lower parts of the castle, then charge up to the roof. Is this not the way the cancer is working? The surgery was supposed to "get it all." Then the radiation was to zap the remainder, but while the radiation team was shelling the bunkers, the bad guys escaped. Now they can go anywhere they please, though they usually stay in the lower body. The dream bulls cannot reach the upper levels of mind and spirit. (According to Dr. Shiller, prostate cancer may progress, rarely, to the lungs, and, very rarely, to the brain.)

The car. It is damaged and must be replaced. The joke is on me. I thought I owned it, but never did. My body, which still seems so young and new, has been damaged. When the time comes to trade it in, I realize I never owned it. The body is something I move around in, but it is not me. I have borrowed it until it is of no use anymore.

The castle. The open courtyard is surrounded by the building. The only way in or out of the courtyard is through the building. The public can view events in the courtyard, but must enter the castle to do so. If the castle is my Self, there is also a public part of me (the courtyard), but even that public part can be experienced only if one "enters in" to who I am. To that extent, what is shown to the public is, in reality, private.

The lower levels, with kitchen, and so on, represent the base (earth-connected) aspects of life. The roof "above," is the mind.

The cupola is important enough that the young warrior and his company want to destroy it, decapitate it; important enough that the children are clinging to it. The bulls can't come up that far. The cupola—the spirit?—is out of their realm. It is the young warrior who attacks it. It is the spirit that breathes life into the children by relieving them of the imprisoning puppet costumes—shades of Pinocchio!

The children. The hope for the future. They will survive only when they "get a life." It is with them that I become engaged in action. Prior to this event, I only observed and tried to stay out of the way, to be safe.

When I told this dream to Cyndi, she pointed out that the Dream Self did three things for the children:

1) It recognized the children.

2) It released them by removing the enslaving puppet costumes.

3) It rescued them by putting their feet on a solid place so they could stand.

The castle may be destroyed, but the children will live. Life does continue.

The father(s). The rational authority, the "adult" of transactional analysis?

My mother. Irma Stegall is the only recognizable "real" person in the dream. Her memory features in the dream right after the pronouncement of death. Mother gave me life and nourished me. She also glorified sickness and death. She had digestive problems as far back as I can remember. Her life centered around her bed and her bathroom. The bathroom, then, is a fitting reminder of my biological mother. The bathroom also symbolizes internal and external cleansing.

The puppet master. The puppet master is as much a slave as are the children. What is his meaning? He tried to fight me off, but I prevailed. Realizing his true role, he became my ally. But who is the puppet master? *The Queen of Hearts.* The archetypal witch commands the battle. She commands by will, not reason. In a deck of cards, the Queen of Hearts has two faces, looking in opposite directions. The *Alice in Wonderland* queen who yells, "Off with their heads!" seems to dominate in the dream. But the "heart" in her name is also important. She *rules* the heart.

The warring armies. Like the two faces of the Queen of Hearts, the two warring armies look and act alike. We don't know which is the establishment and which is the rebel band. While they fight each other, the bulls run amok. Dr. Rick Holmes, my pulmonologist, explained autoimmune deficiency in this manner: The immune system acts like the palace guard, fighting off invading infections and foreign bodies. But it can go haywire and, like the palace guard, start fighting itself. While it fights within itself, infections and foreign bodies can enter unchallenged.

The Young Warrior. In act 1 he is directed by his father, who keeps matters under some control. I do not sense imminent danger. In act 2 he is directed by a woman, perhaps his mother, the "Queen of Hearts."

In act 3 the young warrior becomes a maverick, wreaking his own brand of destruction. But who is he?

I raised that question in a dream seminar. One of the persons present suggested that the young warrior might be my body. Consider: at first the father commands the young warrior, who, in turn, controls the bulls (in other words, the malignancy. All persons constantly produce cancerous cells, but in healthy people the immune system gobbles them up before they can do any harm). Then the queen takes over, commanding him in battle with the rebels against the loyal guard (the immune system?). Then he turns against the house (the Self), trying to destroy the higher levels of mind and spirit.

The waterslide performers. The waterslide surely relates to birth, ejaculation, and/or re-birth. The father establishes the pattern; then the son outdoes him and escapes into the outer (spirit?) world. Is there a relationship of the son to the children in act 3?

The son succeeds by learning from the father, so might he be the obedient alter ego of the rebellious Young Warrior?

※

Emotions in the dream progress from fear to release. In the prologue a kind of terror gripped me that I don't recall having experienced before. In the second part of the prologue, while driving the car, I was boxed in. I drove around and around but never got anywhere. I felt the panic of claustrophobia, similar to the waking panic attacks I have sometimes experienced when I am in a closed area.

In the sequence with the bulls and the young warrior, I moved through a number of emotional states: fascination at the bullfight, anxiety as it entered the castle, anger at the rebellion, urgency in acting to save the children, compassion for their future, relief at their safety.

In the entr'actes, when the show was contained on the stage, I felt contented and amused. Anxiety grabbed me as the performer hurtled off the stage. Relief replaced anxiety when he survived. When the son repeated the act, I felt surprise and exhilaration as he sailed up the aisle and out of the auditorium.

By the epilogue, when I discovered that the car (the shell) I had given up was never mine to start with, I laughed. I thought it was funny. The shell (the body and/or possessions), in the end, was not important.

However, when I returned to the conscious world, body and possessions were still very important!

CHAPTER 20

WHO'S IN CHARGE HERE?

The fall of 1996 approached. We moved into our regular church and school schedule. Fatigue, depression, and panic attacks intensified. On a Wednesday in mid-October, the day before I was to meet Dr. Shiller for the latest PSA results, I could not make myself go to work at school. I started gasping for breath, became dizzy, and starting crying. As I lay on the bed, my whole body went into spasms and started shaking. I finally forced myself to go to school for one voice lesson at 11:00 AM, but sent the others away. After school I managed my afternoon students at the private studio with some sense of normalcy, then met Clarice for our usual pre-rehearsal dinner out. I felt so dizzy and depressed that I asked her to take over the entire rehearsal that evening. When choir convened, I sat back with the tenors while Clarice conducted. Joe, a pharmacologist, noticed my dizziness, shaking, and gasping, not to mention coughing. He suggested that I go outside to collect myself.

Nancy, our pastor, called after we got home that evening. Some choir members had come to her with concerns about my directing of the choir. They felt that something was wrong, that I was not doing the job they expected. I knew it, but did not realize that they could tell.

The next day, before my appointment with Dr. Shiller to get the PSA results, I had to go to the dentist. Dave Morgan, my dentist, is also a personal friend. He refused to do the dental work while I was so badly stressed.

At noon I met Dr. Shiller. When told about the extreme depression and anxiety of the past day, he nodded his head. "We even have a name for it: 'PSA anxiety.'" He had good news, he told us: the PSA was down again, to 36. He then said, "I want to check you down there."

Man, why do you, a urologist, have to use such a bland euphemism for a digital rectal exam? Out loud I just asked, "Why?"

"Well, we didn't do it last time."

"Is there any indication that it's necessary?" I consider the rectal exam to be a highly overrated experience. "I can tell you what you will find. Nothing. When you check for the prostate, it won't be there. You took it out, remember?"

"Well, okay. But next time for sure."

※

Nancy came over to our house that Thursday evening. Clarice and I talked over the church choir concerns with her, then I wrote a letter to the choir.

October 20, 1996. Dear Friends: The time has come for me to give you a full accounting of my health, since it has come to affect my work. When I accepted the position of music director at Saint Andrew, I had no symptoms of ill health. I had been diagnosed with an autoimmune deficiency related to lupus in 1992. With the proper medication, I had experienced no symptoms related to that condition since the summer of 1993.

The diagnosis of prostate cancer was made on June 13, 1995, after I assumed my duties at Saint Andrew. The surgery was July 5, 1995. By the time we resumed choir in August, I was still recovering from the surgery, often feeling tired and not alert. The trauma of the surgery and its aftermath generated a renewal of the symptoms of the autoimmune deficiency: dizziness, depression, shortness of breath, coughing (the condition, which can attack any connective tissue, chose my lungs as its place to camp out). It is possible, though not verifiable, that the autoimmune condition may have even set the body up to be susceptible to the cancer.

When we realized that we were in for the long haul, we got our prayer network in gear. We prayed daily a four-point prayer:

- **believing** that it could drop,
- **specifically**, that the PSA would drop,
- **waiting** for God to act,
- **accepting** whatever outcome God chooses.

I have come to believe that if one attacks illness as a spiritual challenge, the physical outcome is secondary. After all, saintly people have died of the disease, and nonbelievers have survived.

Once the cancer is in the system, it can pop up anywhere, anytime. As a consequence, in spite of my basic optimism, prayers, and support from friends and family, I am acutely aware of the probability of recurrence. Therefore I am resolved to love God completely, and to live fully every day.

So far I have experienced no symptoms that one can identify as being caused by the cancer itself. The only things that have made me feel bad are the treatments! All those factors and more have taken a toll on my energy, emotions, and alertness. Often I can keep going anyhow, but there are days when I cannot force myself to function normally.

As a temporary measure, I request that Clarice take over directing the sanctuary choir, allowing me to take a back seat and serve where I can.

The next Wednesday, after rehearsal, Clarice and I met with the personnel committee, the choir president, several members of the choir, and Nancy. Everyone had already read the letter. They expressed support for both Clarice and me, and accepted without any rancor the changeover. A young attorney, often a clown in rehearsal, leaned forward and poured out, "I can't imagine what you are going through."

I answered, "I hope you never have to."

How did I feel about giving up my position? Relief! At least that is what the rational mind was saying. The subconscious still had some issues to settle.

[Dream, November 29, 1996] For the umpteenth time, I dreamed of directing the choir without my pants on. I had an awful time getting everybody lined up for the processional. There were singers from all our previous choirs. The sanctuary was fan-shaped, with the choir on the left side. I finally got everyone lined up. We processed into the choir loft. As I started to conduct the introit, the attorney-tenor spoke up to remind me that I was not supposed to conduct anymore. It was Clarice's choir now.

Even with daily doses of Zoloft, the emotional swings became more intense. Panic attacks would catch me when I was stooping, bending, going to the bathroom, rushed, or in a small, windowless room. To cope with the panic attack, I would try to find an open space, sit down, and practice deep, slow breathing. However, the least little thing would set the whole process off again. Cyndi suggested I take a complete sabbatical from the church duties.

Dr. Lukowski wanted to put me on higher doses of Zoloft or change to more potent medications. I balked. He referred me to a psychiatric group for evaluation of depression and anxiety medications. The doctor who could make an appointment was Mark Adams, the "new kid on the block" in his practice. My first appointment came on Halloween day, October 31, 1996. Dr. Adams looked like an overgrown choirboy. He was so new to the practice that he did not even have any pictures or plaques on his wall. He turned out to be just the right doctor for me. He confirmed the wisdom of taking a sabbatical.

He reviewed various medications and explained how anxiety functions. Pressing down on the abdominal muscles, as in lifting a heavy weight or forcing a bowel movement, is called the Valsalva maneuver. Two vagus nerves run from the brain stem to most of the organs, including the heart, lungs, and stomach. Locking down the diaphragm will activate the vagus nerves, sending a message back to the brain that one is not getting enough oxygen. The brain sends a message back to get lots of air quickly, so one begins to pant. In a person so predisposed, panic can result. Accompanying sensations may be dizziness and sweating.

Realizing that my dosage of antidepressant was not preventing panic attacks, he prescribed an antianxiety drug, Klonopin. I figured it must be extraordinarily powerful because it comes in 0.5 mg tablets and is listed as a "controlled substance." He prescribed two a day. One day on that dosage and I was in zombieland.

All this jockeying between doctors taught me that although doctors make decisions based on the best evidence and experience they have, they are not omniscient. The patient must take charge of her or his own treatment. I asked Dr. Adams to cut me back to 0.25 mg twice a day. It still caused drowsiness. Then we tried 0.25 mg only at bedtime. Finally I found a dosage I could tolerate.

I decided I could not take off completely from the church duties because Clarice needed me to assist her, to take sectional rehearsals, to lead the tenors (or basses, or occasionally altos), and to play handbells. She was doing so many things for me, I could not take that support away from her.

When I saw Dr. Shiller on November 12, I asked him where we would go if the hormone treatment loses effectiveness. He replied, "We would send you to an oncologist for experimental protocols."

"What kind of 'experimental protocols'?"

He replied that only an oncologist could answer that question.

It sounded to me like it was time to see an oncologist. Dr. Shiller made an appointment for me to see Dr. Kenneth Logan. I got in to see him the next day. It's amazing how a word from the right person can open up space in a full calendar.

Dr. Logan is young, tall, and trim, and doesn't sit down much. He turned out to be a good teacher. For ninety minutes he explained various stages of cancer, the immune system, and types of treatment, filling his handy dry-erase board several times. When he raised the prospect of chemotherapy, I said, "I thought chemo didn't work for prostate cancer."

"That's what we have found in the past. But now we are experimenting with combinations of treatments that may couple hormones with chemo." Among the treatments he mentioned was estramustine, a combination of estrogen and mustard. That's the kind of mustard used in poison gas, like we used against Germany in World War I.

He told me that sometimes, when the PSA gets within a tolerable range, one can opt for a six-month-on, six-month-off routine with treatment. Another choice could be a "drug holiday": go off treatment until the level doubles, then resume. That session with him clarified both the complexity of treatment and the level of control the patient can claim. It was now mid-November, time for another epistle to the medical team:

> After having been run through the gauntlet of specialists regarding my prostate cancer, I decided to pull back and reflect on the treatment possibilities and choices I have encountered. Those treatments and choices are complicated by the pre-existing interstitial lung disease for which I am being treated by a pulmonoloist and a rheumatologist.
>
> But the current treatments are stopgaps. The long-term concerns: It is discouraging to continue a treatment (Lupron and Casodex) that induces depression, anxiety, fatigue, and loss of sex drive. It is also discouraging to realize that its effect is likely to diminish, making more drastic treatment necessary. The primary questions revolve around the balance of quality of life with duration of life.
>
> I understand that the physical effects of orchiectomy and hormone treatment are basically alike. Deprivation of testosterone itself can cause depression. But—the orchiectomy is irreversible. I hold a slim ray of hope in my vision that the malignant activity will reduce to the point that I no longer need to be deprived of testosterone, and that it may rise sufficiently that I can again experience sexual pleasure.
>
> Even with the orchiectomy, continued use of Casodex may be recommended. However, there does not seem to be any convincing study indicating that adding Casodex to Lupron induces longer life expectancy. On the other hand, we do not know whether removal of Casodex would allow the production of enough testosterone to avoid the bad side effects.
>
> At this point, I have three major choices, as articulated by Dr. Logan:
>
> 1) Continue the current program as long as it works,
>
> 2) Drop the Casodex immediately or, if my PSA has dropped to an acceptable level, by the next test on December 20,
>
> 3) Take a "drug holiday." Stop treatment altogether when the PSA reaches a tolerable level, say, below 10.0. (I know, I know! "Acceptable" is below 1.0). Resume treatment only after it doubles.

Because we don't know whether presymptomatic treatment actually increases longevity, I would like to consider the third alternative. If that approach is not feasible, then option two becomes attractive.

If we move into the stage of detectible cancerous growths, I will, of course, want whatever treatments may eliminate the cancer, alleviate pain, or increase quality of life.

I do not wish to undergo treatments that are designed to prolong life at the expense of enjoying the life I have.

My personal beliefs may or may not affect your professional recommendations, but I want you to know that I practice a personal faith in God. I believe that God can, and does, heal disease. I also know that saints die of cancer and that people of no faith get well. Healing can happen on many levels. My fundamental belief is that if disease is approached on a spiritual level, the physical outcome is of secondary, not primary, importance.

You are a first-class team. My thanks to each of you.

CHAPTER 21

THANKSGIVING

Thanksgiving 1996. Joi and Joe had now been engaged for six months. It befell us to go to Joe's house for Thanksgiving dinner with his parents and sister. We all acted clumsy. Lame attempts at conversation fell flat. The weather would not change often enough during our visit to keep talk alive. "The proper way to cook turkey dressing" wore out in ten minutes.

Joe's sister is a veterinarian. She, Joe, and Joi all worked in the same practice. Everybody there was an animal lover. The dogs saved our necks. They gave us nearly an hour's worth of stuff to talk about, if you count all the repetitions about sweet dogs, difficult dogs, big dogs, little dogs, mean dogs, stupid dogs, or whatever other adjectives we could drag out about the world of canines.

Jeremy had driven his own car so he could leave right after we ate. He was a great sport, even giving a gracious, almost eloquent, exit speech. I wanted to leave with him. Because we had exhausted the common subjects—the weather, pets, and how to fix dinner—I wondered: "How can we ever connect with this family? Joe is a fine fellow, but do we have to marry the in-laws, also?"

The means of connection waited a few months before showing itself. I took Joe out to lunch one day the following spring. We talked about all manner of subjects, including the Chicago Bulls, movies, the wedding, and the honeymoon. Then, as I was letting him out at his office, he said, "Tell me all you know about prostate cancer."

"Does your dad have it?"

"Yes. He just found out."

❊

The situation was doubly frightening for Joe's father, Glen, whose older brother had died of prostate cancer when he was in his mid-forties. I felt that I did not know Glen well enough to butt in. I asked Joe if his dad would like me to call and talk with him. Joe thought hard. "I don't think my dad is a very willing or informed patient. Maybe he could call you?" But Glen did not call.

Joe had season tickets to the Indiana Pacers basketball games. For a game with the Chicago Bulls, he got a couple of extras and invited the two dads to go with him and Joi. I was excited because I had never seen Michael Jordan play in person. This also was the first time I had seen Glen since getting the news of his cancer. If we weren't supposed to bring up the disease, it was going to be a long, slow evening. It would be like not talking about the elephant in the room. Then I decided I could not let it go. I got to Joe's house before Glen did. When Glen came in, after the predictable opening banter, I found him alone for a minute. I said, "Glen, I'm sorry about your bad news."

That's all it took. Glen opened up like a dam bursting. He had found out much information from the Internet. Further, he had used the privacy of the computer to say all the things he could not say out loud. Glen and I wound up hugging each other for the first time.

Some time later Joe's sister put on a couples' shower for Joe and Joi. As I walked into the crowd gathered for the shower, I heard, over the conversational buzz, the voice of Joe's mom, trumpeting that Glen was in denial. She proclaimed that he just would not talk about the disease.

I went out to the kitchen and found one of Joe and Joi's work colleagues, a veterinarian, who asked me about my cancer. I filled her in briefly. She said, "You have been in my prayers for months." Being a veterinarian, she likes medical talk, so we went into some detail about treatments. Glen came into the kitchen and stood looking on. The colleague tried to dismiss him, "Oh, Dr. Stegall and I are just talking about some personal things."

I said, "Sue, Glen is in the club. He has prostate cancer, also." So he entered into our conversation. He was lively, probing, informed. He *could not wait* to find someone who would listen and help him deal with his disease!

CHAPTER 22

HOPE IN A NEW YEAR

The new year of 1997 started off in grand fashion with the fifth Lupron shot, this one a three-month dose that charged my insurance company over $1,600. The latest PSA showed a continuing drop, now to 15.7, still quadruple the "safe" level for a man with his prostate, not to mention it was fifteen times what one looks for if the prostate is absent. However, it was a 90 percent drop from the high of 110.5 the previous March. I asked Dr. Shiller to approve dropping the Casodex for three months. He agreed, noting that the PSA had continued its downward trend. I hoped that the freedom from Casodex would ease some of the depression and allow some sexual twinges.

[Journal, January 23, 1997] While I was on my morning walk, the first in a couple of weeks, I tried praying my four-point prayer: belief, petition, listening, accepting. Then I asked, "How do I address you, God? Do I call you 'Father?'" I thought (my childhood friend) Velma was saying something bad when she called her daddy "Father," because Jesus said to call no one "Father" but God. I don't connect with "Jahweh" or "Ground of Being" or "The Wholly Other." How do I communicate with an abstract idea? Jesus called God "Abba" (Daddy). "Allah" is a good name, but it is not in my spiritual culture. I am not at home praying to Jesus, or the Holy Spirit, or to a guardian angel. We try to limit God when we say God needs messengers.

I'm in primary Sunday school. I am seven years old. I draw a dog house, misspelling "D-O-G" as "G-O-D." My teacher is aghast at my "GOD House." But consider: Dog is faithful, will never forsake you, will forgive you, will defend you against harm. Dog—God: not a bad association.

[Dream, January 24, 1997] Clarice, Jeremy, and I were taking an automobile trip with some other people. We made a rest stop. When I came out of the restroom, my car was gone, as were Clarice and Jeremy. Instead, there sat Uncle David's 1956 Chevrolet. I opened the door and looked in. Uncle David was sitting in the driver's seat, but seemed unaware of my presence.

[Observation] Uncle David died in November 1993. In the dream I had died, and my family had gone on and left me to be with him.

After feeling energetic and alert for several weeks, I once again cut the Klonopin to 0.25 mg once daily; then on February 9, I stopped taking it altogether. That move was not a good one. On four consecutive days, from February 20–23, I had major panic attacks. The one on Sunday put me back in bed. I did not go to church. I restarted the Klonopin, but on Monday, the 24th, I got a cold and sinusitis that knocked me out of work for a week.

On the following Saturday, Clarice and I judged the state high school vocal solo-ensemble contest. During the day she reported that her right ear felt stopped up. At dinner she calmly noted, "I would hate to spend Saturday night in the emergency room, but my ear hurts really bad." I took her to MedChek. The helpful young doctor, using what he considered normal first line treatment, prescribed a sulfa drug, in spite of Clarice's telling him she was allergic to sulfa.

She managed, somehow, to play for church the next day, but then became violently ill. It was now her turn to miss a whole week of work.

On Wednesday evening I left Clarice at home and directed the church choir rehearsal. Susan, our children's choir director, readily agreed to accompany us. This rehearsal was the first I had directed since turning the choir over to Clarice in October, five months earlier. Susan did her best at the piano, but could not cope with the Bach cantata[25] we were preparing. I needed her to lead the alto section anyway, so I conducted the cantata from the keyboard. It was an hour of frustration. I have been directing choirs since 1960, my freshman year at Wake Forest. It had always come as second nature, even in my student days. But on this day, I felt out of place, pressured, and scrutinized. Didn't I have the right stuff anymore?

The next morning, getting up was even more difficult than usual. I had an 8:30 voice lesson to teach at Broad Ripple High School. As I walked into the school building, the bowels started pushing. It became a race between the feet and the bowels. The bowels won. I had started taking a spare pair of shorts with me, but I did not have one this time. I cleaned up as best I could, and went up to teach. Meghann, the student scheduled for that hour, was a bright spot in my week. Several times I had arrived at her lessons feeling lousy, only to have her lift my spirits so I could keep going. It did not work this time.

At the next class period, I went across the hall to get the next student. She took one look at me, and said, "Dr. Stegall, you look awful."

"I feel awful." I could not put on.

Another student, as well as the teacher, chimed in. "You look terrible. Go home."

I managed to get myself home, hyperventilating and sobbing part of the way, change into clean clothes, and crawl into bed with Clarice.

I do not remember the rest of the week. I know what my journal and date book tell me I did. I vaguely remember climbing a ladder to clean the gutters of our house, hyperventilating during the whole operation. Otherwise, Thursday, Friday, and Saturday are at best a blur.

On Saturday night, when Clarice and I started our evening prayers, I felt my throat tightening. I thanked God for the blessings we have: each other, our three cherished children, our daughter-in-law, our son-in-law-elect, and Mumzy, for the life she had lived and had given to her daughter. All the time I could feel a great wave building up inside. I started crying. "God, I am sick and tired of feeling sick and tired! I pray that you will take these demons away!" I set into hysterical wailing and sobbing. Clarice held me, rubbed my back, rubbed my legs, talked quietly and soothingly, the voice and touch of my personal angel. After a half hour, we fell asleep, exhausted, in each other's arms.

On Sunday morning we were to present a hymn service at Saint Andrew. Nancy, our interim pastor, wanted me up front leading the hymns. Getting out of bed on Sunday morning generated the usual dizziness and nausea. But by breakfast time, I realized, "I don't feel sick!" The hymn service was a wonderful experience. A rush of energy propelled me up and down the aisles singing,

"See the baby Jesus
layin' in the manger
on Christmas morning
Amen! Amen!"
    —African American Spiritual

For several weeks I felt healthy, alert, and energized. The next PSA, on Friday, March 21, generated no anxiety. Joyce, a college friend of Clarice's who had been in our wedding, called Friday afternoon, largely to check in on us. I found myself telling her that it did not really matter to me what the PSA reading was this time.

Whether it mattered or not, I was excited to receive the news that the PSA registered a scant 6.4. That figure represents a steady decrease from 110 / 67 / 52 / 37 / 15 / 6 since beginning the Lupron and Casodex on March 21, 1996, just over a year before. In my appointment with Dr. Shiller on Thursday, March 27, I requested skipping the Lupron shot. Dr. Shiller pointed out that at the rate we were progressing, in six more months of treatments, we should have the PSA down to maybe 1.5.

I acknowledged that possibility. Then I read off a list of side effects I had lived with for nearly a year:
- fatigue
- depression
- anxiety and panic attacks
- weight gain
- morning sickness
- urinary incontinence
- diarrhea
- hot flashes
- loss of libido
- loss of body hair

I reminded him that one approach to treatment is to go six months on, six months off. If the tendency of prostate cancer is to find, eventually, a source of food other than testosterone, perhaps taking "drug vacations" can delay that change.

Dr. Shiller urged caution. "I must point out the risk of a rapid growth of the cancerous cells. I must point out that your symptoms are not all directly related to the Lupron-Casodex treatment."

I decided that I must listen to what my mind, body, and spirit were trying to tell me. "I am fully aware that the whole process is complicated by the pre-existing autoimmunity for which I have taken Plaquenil since October 1992. I experienced fatigue, depression, and anxiety long before the cancer treatment began. However, I was virtually symptom-free from July 1993 until after my surgery in July 1995. Several of the symptoms, including weight gain, nausea, incontinence, and diarrhea, were major players while I was under radiation. Yet for the few weeks between finishing radiation and beginning hormones in March 1996, I was symptom-free. By April, all symptoms returned in full roar."

I reviewed for Dr. Shiller how those conditions negatively affected my work.

He said, "We are going into uncharted territory."

"I know that. I know the PSA could start rising. Look, Donald, I'm not a fool. I'll take a PSA every month. If it goes up precipitously, we can resume treatments."

He agreed to hold off and watch.

He was right about one important thing. After three months of no treatments, I still tired easily, still experienced depression and anxiety, still got nausea and diarrhea, and still had urinary leakage. I did not lose weight, and my hair did not grow back.

Even so, during those same three months without further treatments, the next two PSA readings dropped to 5.2 and then to 4.7.

Way back when we started the hormones, Dr. Shiller and Dr. Schick had prepared me to expect to gain weight. Already weighing ten pounds more than I wanted to, I did not welcome that prospect. Even so, I could not predict what a trauma it would become when, over the course of a year, I put on an additional fifteen pounds and an extra four inches around the waist.

When I was a child, I was the "fat kid." The peak came in sixth grade, when I was four feet, ten inches tall and 155 pounds, with a thirty-six-inch waist. I heard all the fat jokes. Younger children chased me at recess with sticks and rocks.

I went out for football in high school, promptly lost ten pounds and two notches in my belt, then maintained, with some fluctuation, a thirty-two-inch waist and 155 pounds until I was about forty-five years old. Now, as the hormones did their job, my arms and legs swelled up, and my waist ballooned. I could no longer get my wedding band on. My worst panic attacks came when I tried to get dressed. I got to where I had only two pairs of slacks I could wear. I had grown out of two new suits in as many years. I tried shopping for clothes, but shopping only made matters worse.

One spring Saturday night, Clarice and I went to a local high school to see two of my voice students in their spring musical. Arriving early, we waited in the car until nearly show time. I tuned the radio to *Prairie Home Companion*. Garrison Keillor was presenting a spoof on commercials. This one was a "commercial" for "cat calls" that would deliver various insults to other cats. One of the "cat calls" would say to an unsuspecting cat, "Oh, I see you have no gonads. Is that why you are so obese?" Clarice and I laughed until we cried, then held each other as long as we thought the parking lot security force would let us get away with it, before heading hand in hand, still laughing, into the auditorium.

I finally worked up the nerve to take Clarice clothes shopping with me. I was ready to give up several times, but she always knew one more place to try. We wound up buying several pairs of slacks and several shirts at Sears. When I dressed the next day, I felt relieved that I no longer had to struggle to get the slacks to fasten, and my belly was not bulging the shirt buttons.

CHAPTER 23

_____

WHAT IS SPIRITUAL HEALING?

C ancer does not hear prayer." That is what my physician friend had said. Does it *hear* at all? But who do we pray to? Do we pray to the cancer? Does prayer do anything specific? What is a healing miracle? In the round of doctor appointments in March and April of 1997, I asked each of my team of physicians the same question: "As a physician, what role do you believe the spirit plays in healing?" I let each one determine the meaning of *spirit* according to his own belief system.

The first one I asked is a self-described cynic. His response was, "about 40 percent." He, in his typical fashion, went on to describe his beliefs in negative terms: "I can't cure anyone who doesn't want to be cured."

The rheumatologist would go only so far as to acknowledge that the will to live often sustains a sick person, and that when one spouse dies, the other often follows soon after.

The psychiatrist disclosed that he, not typical of the psychiatric profession, is a firm believer in prayer as a healing agent. He is part of a healing prayer group in his church.

The pulmonologist sees a lot of lung cancer. He told of a recent patient who had wasted away to nothing, and who the doctor thought would be dead shortly. Six months later the man came in, in robust health. "I can only call it a miracle from God." He went on to qualify his statement. He is not particularly religious, but he does believe in the power of God to work beyond human limitations.

The urologist was cautious. Choosing his words carefully, he acknowledged that people recover from illness when there is no rational reason they should.

My dentist, Dave Morgan, sat down by the dentist's chair and expounded for maybe fifteen minutes, waving off his impatient staff as they kept coming in with duties that he needed to take care of. He affirmed miracles, but does not believe that miracles lie outside the natural order. "God created natural order. Why would he violate it? Miracles are events that lie outside our *understanding* of the mind of God."

I asked my daughter. She basically believed that it is a matter of mind over body.

Those answers did not satisfy me. Although I can tune in to each on some level, something is incomplete. Even if one amends the definition of miracle from "events lying outside the natural order" to "events lying outside our understanding of the natural order," we are in a constant retreat. Last year's miracle becomes this year's routine procedure.

I took a closer look at the cynic's backdoor approach: "I can't cure anyone who doesn't want to be cured." If that is the case, what is the corollary? Will healing happen only if you believe enough? If you are not healed, have you failed your test of belief?

My physician friend had said: "People pray and pray, and their cancer keeps growing. Others never pray, and the cancer goes away."

Since I began taking prayer seriously in the 1970s, two ways of thinking had run on parallel paths, occasionally colliding with each other. One said, "Whatever you ask in the name of Christ will be granted to you."

The other jumps out in a camp song: "Let go, and let God have his wonderful way."

A third view, the fatalistic view—"When it's your time, you go; nothing you can do about it"—I have never considered valid.

The battle between petition and submission often raged in my own mind, even as a child. I picked up opposing attitudes from my parents. Daddy would tell of R. G. LeTourneau, a builder of road machinery, who attributed his prosperity to having put his life in God's hands. Mother would subvert that idea when she waxed rhapsodic about some saintly soul who suffered illness and poverty as a witness to God's love. She then tried her best to live up to that ideal.

While I was trying to filter out these questions, I got a chance to witness a miracle firsthand. My Maennerchor friend John Schild called. "I thought you would want to know that George Keene has bladder cancer." George was the kind-hearted soul who had been my taxi driver when needed, and who often called to see how I was getting along. The evening after his surgery, I called his house to leave a message and to let his wife, Kass, know that I was praying for them. To my surprise, Kass answered the phone. "We were so relieved! The doctor got it all!"

"Kass, that is thrilling news!" I did not add that we had thought that my doctor got all of my cancer, but that the cancer had outwitted us. I kept calling periodically. George lost his bladder and his prostate, and had to live with a permanent external urine bag. He said: "It's a bother, but I'm seventy-two. I can handle it."

At a social gathering later, Kass reported a conversation that was nearly identical to the one Clarice and I had the day I found out about my surgery. "George told me that he loves me, and that he knows I love him, but not to be able to show me would break his heart. I told him: 'Love is a lot more than sex. I can live without sex, but I cannot live without love.'"

George's cancer did not go away. Since bladder cancer is different from prostate cancer, the next line of attack was chemotherapy. George, who had been bald for years, joked that the worst part was losing all his hair. He continued to weaken. Then, on May 16, my son Jon's birthday, I got another call from John Schild. "George has come home to die. He knows he doesn't have much time. If you want to see him alive, you need to go right away."

I called immediately, and got George's daughter. She said: "Dad's had a hard day and needs rest. Perhaps tomorrow would be a better time."

On Saturday morning I drove over to George and Kass's house. Cars surrounded the house. Kass was sitting with a friend outside the house, smoking a cigarette. "Carroll, I'm so glad you came. It's been hard on us. We've had the girls here, but George hardly knows anything anymore." She sheepishly held up her cigarette. "See? I've started smoking again!"

Kass led me into the house. George lay on a hospital bed set up in the den so that Kass could work in the kitchen and still be at his side. Their daughters and friends sat around the house. A nurse was near. The hospice chaplain was on his way. One of the daughters said: "He may not recognize you. He sleeps most of the time. Other times he just seems to stare."

I went over to one side of the bed. Kass went to the other. She took his left hand. I took his right hand. "George, it's Carroll. I've come to check on you, young man." His eye strayed in my direction.

"Would it be okay if I sang a song for you?" I started with "Amazing Grace." His eyes focused on my face. A little light seemed to show. Or was it just my imagination? Then I tried "Blessed Assurance." Knowing that George was a rock-solid Lutheran, I asked, "How about, 'A Mighty Fortress'?"

George's eyes never left my face as I tackled the complex text of Luther's great hymn, prompted on occasion by Kass or one of the daughters. Kass was quietly weeping. Tears came to George's eyes. As I finished and let go of his hand, he turned his eyes to her. He tried mightily to raise his right arm up to touch her face. But the arm would not cooperate.

As I turned from the bed, a daughter said, "That's the longest Dad has stayed focused since he came home."

On Monday John called again. "George died Saturday night." I had seen him on his last day. The whole community seemed to converge on Cross and Crown Lutheran Church for the memorial service. I squeezed into a back seat and inadvertently found myself sitting with the choir. John Schild handed me a piece of music. So I got to sing one last time for George. At the close of the service, Kass marched up the aisle, striding beside Pastor Paul, her arms uplifted, her face glowing, singing with the rest of us, "Lift high the cross."

George's family, friends, and church had all prayed for him. All wanted him to recover. Seventy-two was too young for that loving heart to leave us. So where is the miracle? Where is the answer to prayer? I believe George's miracle was that he knew what Martin Luther meant when he wrote: "The body they may kill. God's truth abideth still." Following the memorial service, everyone crowded into the church parlor for a celebratory reception. George was a man who knew how to live until he died. Kass is a woman who knows how to keep living.

After experiencing George's glorious death, I am giving up on trying to define a miracle. I only pray for the eyes to know one when it happens again.

✳

By the spring of 1997, after living with Cyndi's four-point prayer for most of a year, I tried to focus more energy into listening. In our first meeting, back in June 1996, she had prayed for God to support me as I confronted my death. She was the first to cut to the truth. Now, eleven months later, I ran upon this by Saul Alinksky: "Once you accept your own death, all of a sudden you're free to live."[26]

[Journal, May 6, 1997] As much as I would crave protecting my children from disease, failure, pain, heartache, I can't do it. I can't do it physically, and it would not be in their best interests.

I am a child of God. Were God to protect me from disease, failure, pain, heartache, it would not be in my best interests.

I was gradually coming to a new understanding of Jesus's words: "He makes his sun to rise on the evil and on the good, and sends rain on the righteous and on the unrighteous."[27] But faith questions, questions I had thought were settled, rose up again in full battle array. Are illness and calamity punishments for evil? Are they burdens one bears to prove one's piety? Are health and prosperity rewards for good behavior?

Those questions must have weighed more heavily on me than I had realized, for they laid themselves bare in an extraordinarily vivid dream that may be a sequel to the "Bulls" dream recounted earlier:

[Dream, April 18, 1997] I was to be electrocuted. For what crime I did not know. The executioner gave me a choice. I could call it off. I reasoned: "I probably did whatever I'm accused of. I'll die someday anyway. So we may as well get on with it."

Attendants shaved me. They cut open my upper torso at the sternum. They filleted me, taking out my ribs. I saw it. It was just like filleting a fish. I felt no pain. Just wondered what it was all about.

They jellied my wrists, head, legs, and torso. They attached electrodes. I sat in a chair on a stage. People were in the audience. My mind raced as the countdown started.

Ten . . .
"I've got to go sometime, anyway."
Nine . . .
"Let's get this over with."
Eight . . .
"What will it be like to be dead?"
Seven . . .
"What will it be like to die?"
Six . . .
"Will it hurt?"
Five . . .
"What if they only maim me?"
Four . . .
"I'll never hold my child again."
Three . . .
"Wait! I didn't do anything wrong! I'm not going to die for something I didn't do! Stop! I want to live!"

The executioner unshackled me. I tried to stand up, but fell over because I had no ribs. I asked the doctor if they could put my ribs back. He said, "No."

I wondered how I would sing. But I had to try. I propped myself up on a chair and addressed the people in the audience. I said to the people: "I know you all came to watch me die. I believe that most if not all of you came to support me. Those who thought I should be executed didn't bother. But I did not do the thing I'm convicted of. I plan to live until it is the proper time to die. I will take a PSA every month. When the time comes, I will be willing to go.

"I have one request. When you see me, don't ask, 'Oh, how are you?' If I'm having a bad day, I'll tell you. I just don't want my health to be the topic of conversation."

Clarice and I had a baby. I wanted to pick it up, but thought I might drop it because I didn't have any ribs. But I tried, and managed.

Six years after experiencing the Execution Dream, a new ending poked its head out of the sub-conscious:

I picked up the baby.
Held it in my arms.

Look down in its eyes.

The baby's eyes met mine in a steady gaze.

I said, "I'm going to see you graduate from college."

When I told Cyndi that I was puzzled by the filleting of my ribs, she suggested that it might relate to my inability to have an erection. Of course! Bingo! Because I had no ribs, I had trouble standing up. I also thought that I could not pick up the baby, but I could.

Another friend offered this observation: The ribs protect the heart. By "shedding" my ribs, I was exposing my heart.

What does this dream reveal about healing? Let us look first at mind and will. At first my Dream Self acquiesced to the death sentence. It was like Franz Kafka's *The Trial,* in which K. is arrested, tried, and convicted, though charged with no crime. He asks what he is charged with. The judge answers only that he is guilty, the existentialist answer to original sin. My Dream Self faces, as does K., guilt by definition.[28]

An even more powerful dynamic, older than Job, insinuates itself into the Dream Self's mind: "You must have done something wrong. Or else why would you be in this predicament?" Barely in time, the Dream Self's mind and will snap to life. "I didn't do anything wrong! Stop!"

The mind would not accept the absurd falsehoods.

The will asserted the truth and found freedom. Freedom does not guarantee complete recovery.

The body was damaged and weak. The missing ribs could not be replaced. But the body, informed by the mind and emboldened by the will, could learn to continue living with new purpose.

The spirit told the Dream Self that he does not have to be imprisoned by his limitations. He can still produce, and support, new life, as symbolized by the baby.

Clarice also dreamed, the same night, that we had a baby!

The Dream Self's dramatic escape, while intensely personal, is not solitary. The executioner is a kind person who reminds the Dream Self that his life or death is a choice. The executioner seems pleased at the choice for life. The Dream Self has a wife and a child. He is surrounded by friends. The friends do not understand him, but they are willing to accept his choice of whether, and how, to live or die.

Several years ago I wrote a story called "Playing Cowboy." In the story "Sheriff Mike" and "Bandit Ted" get into a shoot-out.

Sheriff Mike got Bandit Ted in his sights. "Pscheoo! Pscheoo! Pscheoo! I got you in the back!"

Ted turned to face him. "Nah, you missed me by a mile."

More shots were exchanged face-to-face at point-blank range. "I shot you four times. You're dead!"

Ted looked Mike square in the eye, then spat on the ground. "I'm not dead 'til I say so."

Whenever I think back on the execution dream, I don't just remember it; I relive it. I see the entire scene in color. I feel helplessness, resignation, fear, indignation, and relief. The dream tells me, on a deep-gut level, that mind and will, body and spirit are intricately intertwined with each other. The Dream Self finds his purpose through his wife, baby, friends, and social environment. The dream tells me that life is a choice that I can joyfully embrace.

Where is God in this dream story?

I believe that God gave me the story, telling me that I have a divine mission. God will give me strength for the mission. The mission will spread beyond me. It will outlive me. But what is the mission? At the time of the execution dream, that mission was just starting to take shape. But after the execution dream, I knew that my mission would involve the healing power of love as I experience it and see it in others.

After this dream I was ready to hit the airwaves.

CHAPTER 24

ON THE AIR

Since 1995 I had been Storyteller-in-Residence at the University of Indianapolis radio station, WICR-FM. Once each month, Paul Irwin Feinman, the convener of the daily live *Indiana Today* program, scheduled a time on the show for him and me to talk about, and tell, stories. Over the years we explored folklore, myth, legends, seasonal stories, family stories, and personal stories.[29]

Early in 1997 I requested that we turn one of our programs over to my experience with prostate cancer. That request touched Paul personally, for he had recently lost a good friend and colleague to prostate cancer. Paul believed that his friend died needlessly, for he had simply waited too long to seek treatment.

Paul reserved the entire hour of my April program to discuss cancer. He wanted to include some guest panelists. As of the Thursday evening before the scheduled program, his producer had run into a string of "no's." So I called my spiritual mentor, Cyndi Alte. "Rev. Alte, I want to make you a radio star! Be sure to wear something loud so it will pick up on the radio!"

Those events that cut deepest into our personal lives are the most universal. Knowing that thousands of others are dealing with similar crises, I did more preparation for this show than for any previous one. Even so, I knew it might be difficult to tell the whole world (or at least the forty-three thousand who listened to that station) about such a personal experience.

Having a trusted friend across the table when we went on the air gave me the assurance I needed. We dealt first with definitions, detection, and treatment.

Paul then turned us to more personal elements when he asked about the role of sexual activity in triggering the cancer. "Should you, or shouldn't you?"

"The more the better!" was my instant reply. "If the seminal fluids build up in the prostate, some irritation can occur. It is better to keep it somewhat depleted."

"Well, that blows one old theory!" Paul exclaimed.

Our discussion throughout was lively, laced with probing questions and with laughter. When Paul tried to get a handle on the stage of my cancer at the present, he asked if the treatments had "gotten it all."

"No. There are still malignant cells in there producing the PSA. We don't know where they are. The potential bad news is that after a while, the cancer may figure out something other than testosterone to feed on, and start growing again."

Paul's eyes popped. He blurted out, "Well, how long do you have?"

I looked right back at him. "How long do you have, Paul? Having cancer is not a death sentence. Being free of cancer does not guarantee immortality. It does not even guarantee that you will live any longer. What we must do is live our lives to the fullest."

At the end of the show, Paul commented on my ability to laugh about something so serious. I replied, "Paul, when I lose my sense of humor, I am dead."

After the show he still had questions, especially concerning how mind, body, and spirit cooperate in holistic healing. Cyndi, pastor and former hospice nurse, is especially attuned to those concerns. Paul asked us to come back for "Prostate Cancer, Part 2" in May.

The following Sunday a retired Saint Andrew choir member came up to me after church. He said he had heard the program. "Are you going to have tapes available? I think that program should be heard by every cancer patient in the country."

On May 18 we reconvened in the little studio on the University of Indianapolis campus. The three of us engaged in such a rich sharing of beliefs, experience, and feelings that I did not much care if anyone else heard it.

We strongly concurred that healing is not a choice among body, mind, or spirit, but a powerful joining of the three. Cyndi pictured it vividly: When spirit, mind, and body are congruent, the person is healthy. But a deviation in any direction can throw the whole system askew.

Paul quoted the well-known sentiment, "God does not give us more than we can handle."

My reply surprised even me: "It is a pretty statement, but I don't buy it. I do not believe that God *gives* troubles to us. Tragedy encroaches on all lives. The response to a catastrophic setback may be ennobling for one person, but debilitating to another."

I do believe, and will stake my life on it, that we can see God in the world around us, in the people we meet, and in the deepest parts of our being. The wonders of nature present us with power and insight when we pay attention. That day in May 1996, when I had observed a live branch growing from a dead, uprooted tree, turned out to be the day that I finally submitted to God's role in rebuilding my life.

CHAPTER 25

REACHING OUT

A fourth dimension completes the essential mind-body-spirit connection. It has been present throughout this chronicle. Now is the time for that fourth dimension to take center stage. In August 1999, I attended a retreat led by John Shea at the Fatima Retreat Center in Indianapolis. Shea, Catholic priest, former seminary professor, teacher of spirituality, author, and advocate of story theology, builds a convincing model for a complete life. The essential elements are the physical, psychological, social, and spiritual. He expands on this paradigm in his book *Gospel Light*.[30] He asserts that the spiritual dimension stands apart from the others. The physical, psychological, and social dimensions can break, but "the spirit doesn't break." The spiritual can inform and strengthen the other dimensions.

After hearing him present those ideas, I cornered him as he lounged in the shade after lunch. "Isn't there another side to that question? Cannot the other dimensions, especially the social, also be conduits to realizing the spiritual?"

His answer was direct. He nodded. "It's a two-way street."

By acknowledging our brokenness—sickness, injury, grief, regret, fear—to another person, we can begin the process of becoming whole. Can we not see our best selves mirrored in a friend who is the face of Christ for us? Then, filled by that loving spirit, will we not pour it out to those we meet? Family, loved ones, and friends can hold us up when we become weak. We, in turn, can support them when they become weak.

Believing it to be time to give something back, I had, in 1998, entered the Stephen Ministry, a nondenominational lay caregiving program. My pre-training interview committee included breast cancer survivor Amee, who by now knew a little of my story. As part of the interview, she had asked, "I suppose you would not want to care for someone who is terminal?"

That question had already come to my mind. "I believe I may have something to give to a person in that situation."

The Stephen Ministry candidates engaged in fifty hours of training before we were commissioned and assigned to care receivers. My assignment was Hal, an eighty-year-old man with lung cancer. In my first visit with him, he joked: "Isn't this a laugh? I quit smoking. Then I got lung cancer!"

We began to visit once a week on the patio of his home. Conversations at first were general, just two people getting acquainted. He loved talking about his children. He loved talking about fishing, golf, and cars. He did not want to talk about his illness.

Finally came the day when he confessed, "I'm just so tired all the time." A year earlier he had been a robust 165 pounds, with a full head of red hair. Now he was down to 130 and bald. He was clearly failing. He was clearly uncomfortable. Yet he sidestepped all the leading questions and other conversation-starting techniques we had practiced in training: "Hal, you say you feel tired. I sense that you are very uncomfortable. Tell me about the chemo you had yesterday."

He changed the subject. "It was rough. Y'know, my daughter called me this morning. It's balmy and seventy-five degrees in California." His daughter, son, and grandchildren checked in on him regularly. The daughter, marketing director for a major national corporation, would call three times a day.

Friends from Saint Andrew would call, drop by, take him out to dinner. After he became homebound, Meals on Wheels kept his body nourished.

He slowed down. He had difficulty taking even the one step up from his den to his kitchen. Chemo made him nauseous. He persistently kept his hurts hidden beneath his hearty demeanor. I decided to break our training rules and divulge some of my experience. When I did, a door swung open. Immediately he opened up to relate his story and feelings. At that moment my health, training, spiritual life, and storytelling experience all converged to open a passage into Hal's inner self. An axiom for storytellers is that we tell our stories to generate stories in others. From the moment of that release, we shared a rich communion. The communion came none too soon.

Two weeks later he went to the hospital. I visited him every day. On a Sunday morning David Liddle, our pastor, asked me to go with him to visit Hal. Hal was in intensive care. His body had shrunk to a near-skeletal state. He did not appear to be conscious.

Made bold by my last visit with George, I took Hal's hand and sang "Amazing Grace" and "Blessed Assurance." David invited the family to join hands with us, then led us in prayer. That night Hal died with his beloved daughter and grandson by his side. I am blessed to have known him for the all-too-short time of three months.

Susan Silberstein, founder of the Center for Advancement in Cancer Education, reports that a constant among cancer survivors is "at least one special healing relationship with a loved one, a health professional, a friend, a support group, or a therapist."[31]

Clarice and I have discovered a network of support that we would never have known had there been no crisis. My work, my family, and my friends are more precious than I could have previously imagined.

Having being led by the spirit to guide a terminal cancer patient to a peaceful death, and having received so much loving care myself, I felt compelled to pursue the next level of caregiving. In April 1999 I attended a national leadership training conference of Stephen Ministry, and became certified to train other people as lay caregivers.

Shortly after completing the training, I talked with a woman whose son was engaged in drugs and in theft. She and her husband had worked hard at being good parents. They had tried tough love. They had tried forgiving love. The daughter, a model of studiousness and responsibility, confided to me that her mom tried to keep up a good front, but cried a lot when she was at home. I called to suggest that the mom seek a

Stephen caregiver. "Laura, I cannot be your lay minister. In this ministry you will be assigned a woman. Also, because we are already friends, I cannot engage in that confidential relationship." We talked for about an hour, during which time she agreed to let me have our referrals coordinator call her. I felt affirmed that this ministry was the right thing for me to do.

The next day I could hardly get out of bed. I fell into a deep depression. When I tried to force myself to get going, I found myself pushing toward a panic attack. The all-too-familiar gasping for breath, dizziness, and their companion delights took over and controlled me.

The same thing happened three more times within a few weeks. I would spend physical and emotional energy working with a person on their problems, then would collapse. I thought, *I am setting a poor example of developing a healthy mind, body, and spirit.*

It required some consultation with my psychiatrist to put a name to what was happening: the physical, social, and psychological factors had become tangled, scrambling messages from the spirit.

The body loses endurance. The body houses the person. It needs to be strong to handle emotional stress. Deprived of testosterone, which is an energy-giving hormone, physical endurance is not going to be as great as it once was, even when one maintains a healthy diet and exercises regularly.

One day I helped my son move some boxes from the basement of our condo. I was soon sweating profusely and gasping for air. He said, "Dad, you're really out of shape." I answered: "I know. I need to exercise more."

My wife asked later, "Did you tell him the main reason you gave out?"

"No. I just didn't think he wanted to hear it."

The emotions become supersensitive. Testosterone deprivation is one factor. Another factor is the necessary unfolding of one's emotions as one deals with the disease. Opening oneself to other people's emotions can in turn shortcut directly to one's own emotions. The constant sense that something sinister is lurking in the bushes waiting to catch one unaware keeps the emotions on edge. I often try to play like life is completely normal. Yet a slight puff of adversity is enough to knock me off balance.

The spirit needs quiet. One must prepare oneself to discover spiritual strength. When one finds a quiet place, both physically and emotionally, the spirit can enter. One can pay a high price for not finding that quiet place.

Soon after beginning to sort out those overlapping forces, I faced an emergency that required my calm strength. The specifics are not important here; the point is that my mind would not cooperate. I had stayed up late the previous night setting up keystroke operations on the computer. Early the next morning, the emergency struck. When I tried to meditate, my brain acted fried:

Control, alt, shift. Find symbols.
"Soon you'd leave me. Off you would go in the mist of day."
Where was I? Oh, yes.
"Be still and know . . ."
Why did this thing have to come up now? . . .
"that I am God. . . ."
Haven't we had enough? . . .
Control, shift, umlaut . . .
Whoa! . . .
"I lift up my eyes . . ."
there's a spider web . . .
"to the hills . . ."
on the window . . .
"and know . . ."
Control, alt, del . . .
Meditation crash.

The spirit may have been knocking on the door, but the mind and emotions were making too much noise to hear. Sometimes that is as close as I can get to "quieting the mind."

The person needs support. Most of us are not made in hermit mode. We need companionship. We need strength that can come from other people. We need to allow ourselves to receive that support with gratitude and without apology. I sometimes try to play the Lone Ranger, taking on another person's burdens when I am not professionally, emotionally, or spiritually equipped to do so.

John Shea identifies the four most important words of spirituality as, "freely receive, freely give." When we give and give without freely receiving spiritual strength, we set ourselves up for burnout and cynicism. When we receive without giving, the gift dries up.

These issues propel me to return to the beginnings of this chronicle. It is time to examine fundamentals. Has the writing helped my own healing? Can it help in healing someone else?

Has it helped my own healing? Louise de Salvo, author of *Writing As a Way of Healing,* is a teacher of writing at Hunter College, in New York.

According to de Salvo, the key elements in writing for healing are (a) events, (b) emotion, and (c) reflection. The writer must engage all three activities for the writing to be therapeutic. Tell (a) what happened, (b) how you felt (or feel) about what happened, and (c) what meaning the experience has for you. De Salvo relates that carrying out such a discipline for a year generated relief from the symptoms of her own severe asthma.[32]

Dr. Joshua Smyth, writing in the *Journal of the American Medical Association*,[33] corroborates her experience. He conducted an experiment in which he had one group of subjects write reflectively about their feelings as they related to significant events (injury, illness, abuse, et cetera) in their lives. A control group wrote about neutral subjects. The group that wrote personal journals showed a marked decrease in symptoms. The control group showed no distinguishable decrease. Several even got worse.[34]

I began my chronicle long before I had heard of de Salvo and Smyth. Yet I have covered events, feelings, and reflections in virtually every aspect of the narrative. On occasion I deliberately have not been explicit regarding my feelings, letting the narrative itself convey the emotion. I affirm with absolute certainty that this process has contributed to my recovery. Clarice also observes that she sees the process as having been therapeutic.

Can it help in healing someone else? Henri Nouwen, in *The Wounded Healer*, writes: "The one who can articulate the movements of his or her inner life, who can give names to one's varied experiences, need no longer be a victim of oneself, but is able slowly and consistently to remove the obstacles that prevent the spirit from entering. . . .

"Only one who is able to articulate her or his own experience can offer oneself to others as a source of clarification. The Christian leader is, therefore, first of all, a person who is willing to put her or his own articulated faith at the disposal of those who ask for help. In this sense one is a servant of servants, because he or she is the first to enter the promised but dangerous land, the first to tell those who are afraid what he or she has seen, heard, and touched."[35]

I continually discover that my experience, while highly personal in its particulars, is universal in its themes. Amee, my friend with breast cancer, read my story. Her response: "I could see myself and my experience in your narrative."

CHAPTER 26

EXPLORING THE UNKNOWN

The effectiveness of hormone treatment is usually around eighteen months. Several unknowns surround the question, "When are you going to use your eighteen months?" Here are some possible scenarios:

• Treat when the PSA rises but you are asymptomatic. Continue until the PSA starts to rise again. When hormone treatment loses its effectiveness, the cancer will resume its growth. This approach keeps the PSA down, but it may not prevent cancer growth. Not all cancer gives off PSA. Also, around 10 percent of prostate cancer cells are hormone resistant.

Unknown: Will the constant treatment escalate the development of resistant cells?

• As in the first scenario, treat when the PSA rises and you are asymptomatic. When the PSA level drops to an acceptable level (theoretically 0.00), stop treatments. When it rises to 20.00, start again. This is the approach that I coaxed Dr. Shiller to try. Though he was reluctant, he permitted it. Gradually some sexual feelings returned.

Unknown: Will the cells learn to be hormone resistant during their "vacation"?

• Treat only when symptoms appear (back pain, swollen lymph nodes, hot spots in bones, and so on), thereby using the eighteen-month effectiveness when it is needed most. Dr. Shiller was unwilling to consider this option, especially since my PSA rose so high so fast.

Unknown: Are hormones actually effective at this advanced stage?

• Instead of hormone treatments, perform bilateral orchiectomy (castration), possibly coupled with Casodex. The basic effect, including side effects, is the same as hormone treatment. All sexual feeling is lost forever.

Unknown: If the testicles are intact, and if the cancer progresses beyond the effective use of testosterone reduction, could sexual feelings return?

The Really Big Unknown: We do not have clear evidence that any of these options prolongs life. None will cure the cancer. If you can't cure and you can't prolong life, the new focus is quality of life: staying in control of such distractions as pain, depression, fatigue, and nausea.

Dr. Bruce Roth, medical oncologist, formerly at the Indiana University Medical Center and now at Johns Hopkins, addressed our support group in 1997. At that time controlled tests to determine answers to the unknowns involved with the various treatment scenarios were just beginning. "Perhaps in five years we will have some answers."[36]

He also pointed out that to detect cancer in one spot, there must be ten billion cells. You cannot detect with one billion. Ten billion cells make a spot that is one centimeter in diameter. Doubling time for prostate cancer cells is measured in years, not months. If you show no detectible recurrence of cancer within five years, you can probably forget about it. According to Dr. Roth, if it takes ten years to show up again, you will be more likely to be "run over by a bus when you are 105 years old" than to die of prostate cancer![37]

In the summer of 1997, we found that my PSA was again on the rise, to 37.99, and then to 46.86. By September, even though I was not convinced of the ultimate need, I agreed to return to the hormone therapy of Lupron shots and Casodex pills. Within a week the all-too-familiar nausea and its compatriots began stirring. But it was different this time. Before the first round of treatments in 1996, the doctors had warned me to prepare for feeling awful. Even so, the side effects had sucked me under before I fully recognized them.

This time I often could recognize the subtle beginnings of symptoms and could take steps to "head 'em off at the pass." I became much more consistent about keeping a healthy diet. My body helped, because by now the sight or smell of a rich pastry or doughnuts made me sick. I'm the one who, as a boy, could eat an even dozen Krispy Kremes between the bakery and home. I also determined to intensify my exercise routine, building up strength before the symptoms erupted. Dr. Adams assisted in rearranging the daily pill-taking routine so that three or four stomach-irritating drugs would not hit at the same time.

From the August 1997 PSA high of 46.86, the next reading in November registered 7.86, the greatest percentage drop since beginning the hormone treatments. By April 1998 it was 4.3, the lowest count since I had begun radiation in November 1995. In September 1998 we stopped the treatments again. The PSA continued dropping to a low of 1.07 in January 1999. Dr. Shiller was amazed. He said, "That's the reason medicine is an art, not a science."

By March it had risen to 4.55, but I figured, *I lived with 110.5; I can live with this,* and opted to remain off the treatments.

Even then the demons of depression, anxiety, incontinence, diarrhea, and fatigue stayed with me. The sex drive did not return. I thought again, *Why not go ahead and have the orchiectomy? All the testosterone has been killed off anyway.* Then one Saturday night in April, the libido charged in like a roaring lion. It took seven months for sexual feeling to return. When I had gone off treatments, only three months had elapsed. *The system is definitely slowing down, but I'm not yet willing to kill it off.*

The search for clear answers to treatment effectiveness continues. The *Journal of the American Medical Association (JAMA)* reported studies that address questions regarding the most effective use of hormones and other treatments. Howard I. Scher, MD, writes in *JAMA,* May 5, 1999:

The objectives of treating a rising PSA level are to prevent metastases, symptoms, or death due to prostate cancer. Central to this approach is the ability to define and to redefine continually the prognosis of patients as the natural and treated course of their disease unfolds. Not all patients with relapsing disease have an equal risk of death due to prostate cancer, and only some will develop clinical metastatic disease or symptoms of disease in their lifetimes. Do all need immediate intervention? No. Do all need any treatment? No.

For most patients, the long-term effects of impotence, hot flashes, gynecomastia [breast enlargement], anemia, weakness, fatigue, muscle wasting, and accelerated bone loss with possible osteoporotic collapse do not justify an uncertain level of benefit. The situation may be different for a patient at high risk for the early development of metastatic disease. Trials to address the question are ongoing. At this point, however, patients can only be informed of the potential benefits and the recognized adverse effects of medical castration. To date no cytotoxic [cell-destroying] approach has been shown in a randomized trial to improve survival.[38]

A 1998 study by Anthony V. D'Amica, MD, PhD, et al., describes well-differentiated disease (Gleason score of 2-4), moderately differentiated disease (Gleason score of 5-6), and poorly differentiated disease (Gleason score of 7-10), where 2 indicates barely discernable cancer and 10 means the prostate is full of cancer. The study deals principally with the effectiveness of brachytherapy (radioactive pellet implants), cryosurgery (freezing with liquid nitrogen), and prostatectomy, all cytotoxic treatments. It does not consider hormone treatments. It points to the same uncertainties encountered by Scher.

"Men with moderately differentiated disease (Gleason scores of 5-6) face a modest risk of death from prostate cancer that increases slowly over at least fifteen years of follow-up. These men face a risk of dying from prostate cancer, but it is unclear from a population perspective what percentage of these men will actually benefit from treatment."[39]

Thus we now know little more about long-term effects than we did when I started treatments in 1995.

Dr. Shiller was shaking his head as he walked into the examining room. He was reading my chart. It was early July 1999. "Well, your PSA is down again. It's been a year since you had treatments, and the reading has dropped from 4.55 to 3.55 since April. Considering where you've come from, that's really good." This appointment had generated a lot of anxiety. The last time I had gone off hormones, the PSA had dropped, then shot up dramatically, requiring a return to treatments. This time it had arched up a little, then dipped again.

For the first time since beginning treatments, I felt free.

A couple of weeks later, I saw my primary physician. When I reminded him of the drop in my PSA, his response was: "I think we ought to get down on our knees and thank the good Lord. You must have done something right. I believe you have beat the odds and conquered this thing."

What am I hearing? This is the doctor who is a self-described cynic. "Jack, I can't believe you are advocating prayer."

"Why? I'm not a member of any organized religion, but I am a very religious person." In ten years of treating me, he had never let on.

I make no claim to having "conquered this thing." The final results are not in my control. Besides, I have an old habit that haunts me. Many times I have found myself saying, "Things are going pretty good," only to be knocked down. For years I lived like a hockey puck. I went smoothly in a straight line until something else whapped me and sent me sailing off in another direction. Now I am learning to be more prepared for the unknown.

My dear friend Susan, the Professional Pessimist, says, "There's one good thing about being a pessimist: you're never disappointed."

I, the Eternal Optimist, counter, "Oh, yes! A pessimist is disappointed when things go right!"

She comes back swinging. "No, when things go right, then it's a pleasant surprise."

I found a greeting card that was perfect for her. It read, "A positive attitude may not solve all your problems . . . but it will annoy enough people to make it worth the effort!"

But that is not the level of hope, or lack of hope, I now live with. "Sody Salaraytus," that country tale I dealt with earlier, holds the key: The reward is strength to keep living! The reward is not knowing what will happen, yet living with the assurance articulated best by St. Paul:

I am convinced that
neither death, nor life,
nor angels, nor rulers,
nor things present,
nor things to come,
nor powers, nor height,
nor depth, nor anything
else in all creation,
will be able to separate us from the love of God
in Christ Jesus our lord.[40]

Research into the nature of the disease, and into treatments, keeps turning up new challenges. Instead of closing in on one central cause and cure, each new discovery seems to open new avenues of research. My physicians have as many questions as they have answers. It would be foolish for a layman to try to presume to have definitive answers. By the time this chronicle goes into print, new studies will have been done, new discoveries made, tried-and-true treatments discarded. I have researched current treatment options as far as my layman's brain will go, but make no pretense of this being a comprehensive medical guide. It is, instead, one man's attempt to understand what is happening to him.

One may not control the course of a chronic disease. One can, however, control one's response to the disease. Disease, like death and separation, can produce shock, denial, despair, anger, and self-pity. How does one move out of shock and into action? How does one move out of denial into affirmation? How does one move out of despair into hope? How does one move out of anger into love? How does one move out of self-pity into compassion?

I cannot dictate how another person must find strength. I only know that I have looked for strength and found it everywhere: in nature, music, books, friends, family, and faith in God. Even in a rotting maple tree. It is a constant renewal. Every day is a new challenge and a new chance.

At the end of July 1999, Clarice and I attended the annual church music workshop, seeing again our once-a-year friends who have shared so many of our trials.

One of the first persons I spotted was Beth, who had asked me two years earlier if I was having PMS "the way the rest of us do."

I gave her a big hug, and said, clearly within Clarice's earshot, "Come talk to me, you gorgeous hunk of femininity!"

Then she batted her eyes at me, pulled me close, and said, "Okay, how are you doing, really? Cut the bullshit and give it to me straight."

My response, not uncharacteristically, was to tell a story. "I heard a piece on the radio recently about a village in southern Mexico that sits on the side of a volcano. About ten years ago, the volcano became active. Seismologists predict that sometime in the next thousand years, the volcano will blow."

She picked right up on it. "So it could erupt next week, or it could not happen in a lifetime. You just never know."

"That's how I feel. I'm living with a volcano that may blow anytime, or may never do anything. It's always there. I can never get away from it. I still have depression and anxiety to deal with. I tire easily. I have an upset stomach every morning. You wanted it raw, without the bullshit. So you got it."

This conversation may sound like I have lost my optimism. Not at all. But one must acknowledge all facets of one's experience. Jungian psychologist Christina Middlebrook, in *Seeing the Crab,* puts it, with her blunt eloquence, this way:

> I've been through a lot, fighting this disease. I need the proof, my war wounds, my badges of honor. In the beginning, reeling from the shock, when I felt drowned in information that threatened to swamp all of life as I had known it, even then I said I had to get to know this cancer, this vile crab, and make it part of who I am. . . .
>
> Jungians are determined to acknowledge the shadowy side of life. I have a colleague who consulted once in a nursery school where the children were having considerable nightmares. When she discovered that the teachers (and parents, at the teachers' suggestion) were editing out the evil characters and frightening endings from the fairytales and nursery rhymes that they read aloud, my colleague told them to stop.
>
> "Read these classics as they were written," she instructed. "Don't interfere with myths that have endured for centuries."
>
> The children's nightmares subsided.[41]

Tuesdays with Morrie reveals exceptional insights in Mitch Albom's interviews with his dying former professor, Morrie Schwartz. Morrie insisted,

> By throwing yourself into these emotions, by allowing yourself to dive in, all the way, over your head even, you experience them fully and completely. You know what pain is. You know what love is. You know what grief is. And only then can you say, "All right. I have experienced that emotion. I recognize that emotion. Now I need to detach from that emotion for a moment."

Morrie stopped and looked me over, perhaps to make sure I was getting this right. "I know you think this is just about dying," he said, "but it's like I keep telling you. When you learn how to die, you learn how to live."[42]

I would never ask for disease. But I got it anyway. It is not the worst thing that can happen. It is nothing like it would be if I were to lose one of my children or my wife. The disease may eventually take my life. If it doesn't, we have an ironclad guarantee: something else will. By confronting the inevitability of death, I realize how much I love life.

My resolve is to treat every day as a gift and to leave the future to God. Through this process I have been able to refine my own mission statement:

To cultivate a healthy mind, body, and spirit.

To encourage others in their own journey toward wholeness.

CHAPTER 27

THE JOURNEY BECOMES A QUEST

A s the summer of 1999 moved into fall and another year of teaching routine, indications of cancerous activity had been negligible for over a year. It was time to take on some new commitments. I volunteered to lead a Bible study using Marcus Borg's challenging book on the historical Jesus, *Meeting Jesus Again for the First Time*.[43] The study absorbed me to the point that Clarice started calling it an obsession.

The questions "Who was the historical Jesus? What really powered the beginning of the Church? What does that man have to do with my life?" raised their heads and shouted at me. It was while researching the Bible study that I attended the retreat with John Shea, mentioned earlier. In that retreat Shea led us to contemplate the stories of Jesus as they speak directly to us. Historical context was not really in the equation. On the Saturday afternoon that I found John lounging in a recliner under a shade tree, I asked my burning question, "How important is the study of the historical Jesus?"

He answered, "I taught Quest of the Historical Jesus for twenty years in seminary. I have come to believe that the closer we get to the historical Jesus, the further removed we become from the Christ of faith."

That conversation shifted the emphasis of my study. It became more than a strictly historical investigation. It became a quest for the spiritual foundations of Christianity. It became a quest to discover what has sustained persons of faith over thousands of years. It became a quest for the meaning of my own life.

✳

David Morgan was my voice student before he was my dentist. In 1988 we had been living in Indianapolis for less than a year, and we had not yet found a family dentist. One afternoon a lower right molar began to throb. At first I felt pressure rather than pain. By late evening I decided I could not wait for relief. I knew Dave was a pediatric dentist, yet he was the only dentist I knew. Around 9:30 I called him at home. "Dave, when is the earliest tomorrow morning I can call your office for an appointment?"

"What is bothering you?"

I described the throbbing pain and swelling gum.

"Meet me at my office in a half hour. Have someone drive you. You won't be able to drive home." Jon drove over with me, and waited while Dave opened up the clinic for a private show.

Working from 10:00 until midnight, he performed a root canal treatment and told me to come back at 9:00 AM. The next morning his deep bass voice was particularly grave. "If we had not done that work last night, by this morning your jaw would have been swollen like a tennis ball."

He took X rays and performed a thorough checkup. What he found in my mouth was a gold mine for him. My teeth were crumbling, leaving no foundation for aging fillings. He set up a plan to rebuild my mouth, replacing all my teeth with crowns. The top he finished in 1997. Two years later deterioration of the lowers meant the time had come to tackle them.

On August 17, 1999, I reported to what has become "the Stegall Chair" in Dr. Morgan's office for a five-hour crown preparation. Because he was going to have to cut deep, and because the procedure would take so long, he gave me nitrous oxide. I have long been able to go to sleep in the dentist's chair. I drifted in and out of sleep for a couple of hours.

About the third hour, I thought, "I ought to do something worthwhile during my hours of confinement." I shifted into a meditation mode, silently reciting from Psalm 46:10, inhaling slowly and deeply silently exhaling the words:

Be still / and know / that I am God

Be still / and know / that I am

Be still / and know

Be still

Be.[44]

After several repetitions of the mantra, these silent words emerged: *Lord Jesus Christ, reveal to me your true nature.*

The thought was hardly complete when I "heard," *"You have said it."*

Immediately my rational, skeptical brain was on the attack. *What do you mean, "You have said it?" Those aren't even words I use! I don't pray to Jesus. I think it's presumptuous. I pray to God. I honor Jesus. "Lord Jesus Christ" is a traditional address I don't use.*

"Listen to yourself."

Okay, okay! What do those words really mean?

Lord—master, teacher, leader, guide, mentor—the one to whom I give my loyalty.

Jesus—Yeshua, the Jew from Nazareth, ca. 4 BCE–30 CE; itinerant preacher, healer, exorcist, challenger of conventional wisdom—the one who shows me, by his humanity, the nature of God.

Christ—Cristos, Messiah, Anointed One, Son of God—the one chosen by God to reveal divine nature to humans.

What does it mean that a historic form of address I have studiously avoided leaps out to claim my total attention?

Thoughts of this nature swam through my consciousness as Dave drilled and hacked at my teeth. I was still busy with my inner thoughts when Dave turned the nitrous down and began feeding me pure oxygen. I wanted to yell at him: "Wait! Leave me under a while longer! I'm on the verge of a eureka!"

The next morning I tried to bring some shape to those thoughts as I wrote in my journal. John Shea had suggested some criteria for determining the truth of an experience. I subjected my inner encounter of the previous day to those criteria:

• *Is it self-authenticating?* Does it ring true? Does it enlighten? Does it have authority? Does it say, in the words of that great philosopher Popeye, "I yam what I yam"? I had prayed, spontaneously, the kind of prayer I would not pray if I were planning it out. I am very careful with language. I have constructed a rational argument for not praying to Jesus. Yet that is precisely what flowed out, natural, clear, and unpolluted. So if I struck the rock against my rational constructions and pure water flowed out, then the experience is self-authenticating. It needs no other substantiation to prove it is real. "One thing I do know, that though I was blind, now I see."[45]

• *Does it put you in a mode of service to that truth?* Yes. It demands to be shared. It shaped my whole approach to the Bible study.

• *Does the receiver possess it?* No. This is not my creative imagination or intellectual construction. It snuck up on me with a truth validated by millions over millennia, a truth my intellect mulled over but resisted. "You made me love you—I didn't wanna do it."[46] It becomes a part of me, but as a gift, not as an earned possession.

• *Is it free of my ego?* Yes. The experience is its own witness. It demands to be shared. It subverted my rational constructions. My ego did not create the experience. Nor did my intellect, will, or imagination. Serene confidence that the experience is real and demands to be shared allows me to tell it, and live it, without being self-promoting. But I know this is a dangerous land for me. Feigned humility is a frightful false god.

• *Does the experience push me back into the physical world?*

I guess that means my feet will have to do the talking!

Shea: "Your passion may be God. God's passion is the earth."

The Shakers say it well: "Hands to work; hearts to God."

Likewise the Zen axiom: "First enlightenment; then the laundry."

Sharing such an experience can be hazardous. That moment of enlightenment was intimately tied to our Bible study. When I shared it with the Bible study group, people went mute, shifted in their chairs, and studied the carpet patterns. Elaine, silver-haired, witty, very proper, has learned and observed much in her eighty years. She broke the silence. "You better watch out for that nitrous! It can mess with your brain."

❋

Early in October another troubling dream visited me:

Uncle David had died. In his workshop a window had broken out years ago. No matter how many times he repaired it, it always shattered again, allowing arctic air to blow throughout the summer as well as in the winter. Aunt Marjorie took me through the workshop, urging me to hurry and not to look either left or right. But I could not help myself. I felt the icy wind rushing through the broken window. The window beside it was intact, but shattered glass lay all around on the floor in front of the broken window. Besides, the shade would not stay down. I saw holes in the shade where Uncle David had nailed it down, only to have it rip out again.

Uncle David's circular saw lay on the workbench. As I walked past, the saw swiveled toward me. The sheath was off the blade. The blade aimed directly at me. I thought, "The wind caught it." I took a step backward. The saw turned. No matter how I moved, it swiveled so the blade pointed directly at me.

Aunt Marjorie hurried me out of the room. She explained that once, when Uncle David was using the saw, it had turned itself toward him. He had thrown it down on the table and unplugged it. He never went near the saw again, but whenever he went through the room it would always point its blade toward him.

In the following days, I expanded on the dream, developing it into a short story titled "Grandpa's Saw." It seemed like a good spook tale for my monthly radio show. A couple of weeks later, my storytelling friend Ellen hosted an intimate October gathering of storytellers to visit, to talk about storytelling, and to swap spooky tales. Bob Sander, the founder of Storytelling Arts of Indiana, was among the group of friends gathered at Ellen's house that evening. I decided to give the story a trial run. Storytellers make a wonderfully receptive audience. As a species they do not display the pettiness and jealousies I have grown accustomed to in *artistes*. They are keen in perceptions. They are honest.

As we were leaving Ellen's house, I told Bob the dream basis of the story. When I had told the story that evening, I had described the saw blade as aiming at my chest. But the moment I gave that description, I remembered—in the dream it was aimed at my groin! Then it all made sense. The broken window that could not be repaired or covered up, the constant chill, the ever-threatening machine that turned on of its own volition: everything spoke of physical, emotional, and spiritual anxieties that would not go away.

When I got home, there was a message from Bob on my answering machine. I called him immediately. He said: "I've been thinking about your story. It seems to ring true to the experience of cancer patients. I think you could seriously consider sharing that story with other people with cancer."

In further reflection I have realized that Uncle David, who died in November 1993, and Aunt Marjorie, who died in the spring of 1994, have entered my subconscious as not just themselves but as archetypal ancestors. Their farm and their simple life were a source of childhood stability for me as we moved our own residence from town to town. They were the last living persons of their generation. Once they were gone, I had no physical links to my family history.

But they entered my dreams as warnings, as guides, as comforters. I am not the only one to be thus affected. Their daughter and my closest cousin, Phyllis, told me that on the day after Uncle David died, Aunt Marjorie "took sick," went to the hospital, and never left. On the night before Aunt Marjorie died, Phyllis dreamed that Uncle David drove up in his 1956 Chevrolet to pick up Aunt Marjorie and take her home. That was the same car I had seen him in during my earlier dream about dying.[47]

Those spiritual events and dreams were preparing me for the next stage of my cancer encounter. I had grown a little complacent, as well as self-conscious about even talking about my cancer, because it seemed no longer to be much of a factor in my life. PSA levels had stayed low for eighteen months, prompting Dr. Lukowski's surprise affirmation, "You have beat the odds and licked this thing."

In addition to the Bible study, another major project claimed my attention. Lee Jones, a longtime musician friend, leads a woodwind quintet. A number of years earlier, we had heard a recording of Lewis Carroll's *Alice in Wonderland,* set to woodwind music by American composer Alec Wilder, with narrative by British actor Cyril Richard. For twenty years Lee had wanted to bring it to the stage. He asked me to edit the text, narrate, and sing in a one-hour concert version.

We did three performances in November, 1999, which we believe are the first-ever live performances of this music. Our show can best be described as a one-man reader's theater with music, props, and audience interaction. Lee, the quintet, and I were all excited about bringing this near-forgotten music to the stage. All the while I kept getting socked with depression and fatigue.

Seven days of depression. Swimming against a strong undertow. Part of the time I swam along on the surface with little effort. Then the undertow would grab me and pull me under. I would force myself to the surface, gasping for air. Then the current would grab me again. So—"normal" was keeping my head out of the water. [48]

Our second performance of *Alice,* at an elementary school, caught me in the middle of that depression. I could barely get out of bed that morning. I had cancelled all other appointments for the day so I could concentrate on mental preparation. I had edited ruthlessly to cut the sixty-minute story down to forty-five. Susan (the professional pessimist. I like to call her *mi amica Susanna*) had arranged the school performance, and had lined up children to assist me at critical places.

For this performance I took on the responsibility not only for props, carrying the narrative, and being in voice for the songs, but also for pacing the program, cueing the children for their walk-ons, and making sure we ended in time for the children to catch their school buses. I unloaded all my equipment mid-morning, left to attend a funeral, grabbed lunch, and rushed back to the school to set up for the concert. I began to feel panic grabbing me. I had to force myself to get ready for the onslaught of three hundred children.

By the time the children began filing into the gym, however, adrenalin took over. I could feel the emotional charger shoot up to performance mode. I intermingled with the arriving children, telling them, group by group, what to expect, and teaching them the signals for audience interaction, just like I had done so many times before. One of the instrumentalists, seeing the orderly army of children coming in, whistled under his breath: "This is going to be tough. But—you're the pro at this. You're used to it, aren't you?"

"Yep. Done it lots of times," I shot back. But always when I was in complete charge. When I do a storytelling program, I can stretch stories when children respond, cut stories short when children get restless, add others, or delete on the spot. When I had instrumentalists and child supporting actors to cue, I was a prisoner of the script.

The children proved to be a wonderful audience. After we got into the rhythm of the performance, we were having such a great time that I spontaneously turned the "Caucus Race" into a real race with a half-dozen children. For the "Pig and Pepper" chapter, I led the audience in a sneezing and wailing contest.

When we were about half done, Susan sidled up to me. "You've got ten minutes." Where had the time gone? We were supposed to have forty-five minutes. I held a hasty whispered conference with the players, telling them to cut three musical pieces and a whole chapter of dialogue. By pushing the narrative to "rain tempo" (a term from outdoor theater, meaning "get it over with before the storm hits"), we managed to finish just as the buses were pulling up in front of the school.

I went home and collapsed. I confessed to Clarice that maybe I no longer had the emotional stamina to work under that pressure. Maybe I should call it quits.

Our last performance, at a retirement center, was fun and well received. I felt relaxed and in control. I put my out-to-pasture thoughts away.

I did, however, request that Dr. Adams change my medication. We began the transition from Zoloft to Prozac. Dr. Adams told me, "It is a little stronger than Zoloft in generating energy, but that same effect could increase anxiety. So we better stay with Klonopin to alleviate anxiety."

I read that Prozac can encourage amnesia. Because I am already the quintessential absent-minded professor, I don't need any help forgetting. Using Prozac can lead to decreased sexual function. Big deal. I'd been nonfunctioning for four years already.

The first week was hell. The second week depression and anxiety still kept hitting. The third week I began to feel energetic. Exercising became a pleasure again. I stopped having that "how–can–I–make–it–another step" fatigue. I would need that energy, and more, for the week that lay ahead.

CHAPTER 28

WHERE ARE WE GOING?

On December 14 my spiritual mentor, Cyndi, had surgery for breast cancer. Although she had been able to guide me to a peaceful acceptance of my situation, when it hit her, it hit hard. Clarice and I were among the first persons she called to let us know her diagnosis and treatment plan. She was frightened and distraught. Now it was my turn to pray for her. That morning my main thoughts were for Cyndi, her husband, Doug, and her family. Her church gave her a paid leave for as long as she needed to recover. Her surgery would be major enough that she planned to be off of work for about six weeks.

That same day my women's chorus had a holiday luncheon. Before the luncheon I dutifully showed up at Dr. Shiller's office for my six-month checkup. He strode into the examining room. He wore one of the new faddish iridescent shirts, in lavender, with a matching lavender tie, under his starched white jacket. His voice was as hearty as ever, but he didn't smile and he didn't look at me. His eye was on the chart. "Well, it looks like the PSA is up. It's seven—"

That's okay. I have already decided not to do anything if it's below twenty .

"*Seven-ty* point nine seven."

Yikes! That blows my whole plan of action.

I forgot my determination to take charge of my own treatment. I was mute as he ordered the new plan of attack. "We're going to start you back on the Lupron shots and the daily Casodex pills. I'm also ordering some blood work to check your hemoglobin, liver function, and so on. Next week I want you to check into the lab for a bone scan. If we find hot spots, we can radiate them to give you some relief. It is possible, though not likely, that the cancer can eat through the bone, actually causing lesions in the bone."

He's laying out major battle plans here. I told him, "My stomach is churning, but I am listening and will do everything you ask." *This is not a time for "what ifs."*

Immediately I went to the lab for the blood draws, then drove up one block to the pharmacy to get the prescription filled.

"Mr. Stegall, do you have a new insurance card?"

"No, not since January."

"Well, our screen is saying that your old card is invalid. Your insurance has been cancelled."

I exploded. "What?" This was a new pharmacist. "That can't be!" I had never seen her before. "This is an error! A clerical error that was to have been solved three months ago!" And I was yelling at her. Seeing her stricken look, I calmed down a little. "I'm yelling at you, but it's not your problem. Indianapolis Public Schools messed up. But no way can I pay for a three-hundred-dollar prescription out of pocket." I had to leave empty-handed.

There was still the luncheon to attend. I got to the luncheon a half hour late. This was a big, once-a-year event for the women's chorus. My arrival was greeted by many solicitous "we-were-getting-worried-about-you's." I told them part of the truth. I simply said that a doctor's appointment had taken longer than I had scheduled. Women, especially those over fifty, know all about doctors. No further explanation was asked for. The hostess, dressed in an elegant cream-colored pants suit with gold trim, looking fresh and much younger than her sixty-five years in hardly any makeup, brought me right into the thick of the party. Her ten-thousand-square-foot home with a thirty-foot-high great room ceiling not only generated the expected gasps and sighs; it also was welcoming and comfortable. I looked around at the people who were gathered. I had been directing this group for six years. Clarice had directed them for two-and-a-half years before that. I knew about their cancer, lupus, and diabetes; sick and unemployed spouses; sons who died of epilepsy and suicide; divorced or divorcing daughters; parents with crippling arthritis or Alzheimer's.

"There but for the grace of God go I?" That sentiment is bull hockey. How can I look at another person's trials, and thank God for not being that person? We are all in this together. I am not an isolated or unique case. I learn from others who go before me and along with me. They show me how to handle adversity.

I did not give a medical report. Even so, they surrounded me with a warmth that reminded me to embrace all life experience, because all experience shapes who we become. When I related this experience to Clarice, she reiterated what she had said a couple of times before: "You have no idea how much those ladies love you."

Now it was off to the battleground to fight about insurance. The next morning, I told my boss, Ralph, the director of the Center for Performing and Visual Arts at Broad Ripple High School, about the insurance news the pharmacist had sprung on me. Now it was his turn to yell. "They can't do that! It's illegal to drop you without notification. Besides, I was assured that your coverage was corrected."

I had gone to bat for him, very publicly, when his job had been threatened two years earlier. During that time our mutual respect had blossomed. I knew he was not giving me the runaround. By Thursday he could give me no new assurance. "I've done all I can do. You have to carry the ball now."

I nearly lost all my fragilely wrapped composure right there in the main hall at Broad Ripple High School. "Ralph, I don't think I can take much more."

That night I had another storytelling program to present, this time for a club Christmas party. The lady who invited me said, "Now, Carroll, I want it funny. I want it Christmas. Risqué is okay."

"Jackie," I had countered. "I can do Christmas. I can do funny. But risqué? I don't do risqué." I wrote a new story called "A Christmas Pageant Nobody Would Ever Forget." It focused on mischievous ten-year-old boys who deliberately sabotaged "We Three Kings." I had done a sketch from it for my December radio show. Paul, the host, thought it was really funny. A trial run of the full story on Tuesday at the luncheon got some good laughs, but also told me that I needed to do some major editing.

With Cyndi's surgery, my PSA news, the battery of tests, and fighting city hall over my insurance, my time and energy were not focused on the story. I was straining my emotional limits.

The club treated Clarice and me to dinner. We got there late, but a high school show choir was on before me, so we had plenty of time to eat. Jackie told me to take as much time as I liked—up to thirty or forty minutes.

"The high school group has a half hour. Then the president has a few announcements. After that, it's all yours."

The club president got up. He was sorting through a sheaf of papers. Instead of adjusting the mike stand to his height, he leaned over it, scrunched over sideways. He rambled on with club business for a half hour. People started getting up to go to the restroom. I went around to Jackie and said: "What do we do? Before he finishes, half the people will have left and the other half will be asleep!"

She said, "Can you cut it really short?"

"Not and do this story. But I'll do my best."

The president shuffled through his papers to find the bio sheet I had given him. He couldn't pronounce my name. "We've never had a story-teller before, but here's a good one I just heard." He tried out a lame joke.

I could not think quickly enough to change to another story. I never use notes and I had not lived with the new story long enough to make intelligent cuts.

I bombed.

I don't recall another time in my storytelling career when I would come flat out and say that. Clarice did not argue with my evaluation.

Friday I spent most of the day at the education administration offices downtown, trying, in vain, to find someone who could even converse intelligently about the school's insurance provisions. Those who did know anything were "unavailable."

Saturday night, at Clarice's office dinner dance, I was rude to two people. I went out of my way to encounter them. I don't do things like that. Anybody who claims that testosterone deprivation makes one docile should just try it for a while.

Sunday our church choir presented its Advent choral service. Thank God, something went right. The pastor thought it was wonderful. The congregation went away jubilant. The choir was affirmed and fulfilled. They also gave Clarice and me a very generous gift certificate, far more than they had ever given us before.

Monday I was back in battle gear with the education administration. At my insistence, the two people who knew anything about the original error and could do something about it, but who would not see me the previous Friday, met with me in a three-way conference. No one would admit to the error. However, they would agree that "an error had been made." They arranged to restore my full health coverage, retroactively, with no penalty and no reapplication. Everything I wanted; everything that had been promised three months earlier. But I had to have that assurance in writing before I could proceed with the prescribed medication and with the scheduled bone scan.

Where had my carefully thought out psychological-physical-spiritual-social balance been? On a wild run on a rickety roller coaster with loose wheels.

Every day requires the same efforts. Every day is a new beginning. Many mornings, especially when under pressure, I would feel nauseous. If I forgot, ignored, or "didn't have time for" meditation, prayer, exercise, a decent diet, and positive human contact, the undercurrent could drown me.

I planned to paint our home music room during Christmas vacation. The room had previously been a nursery. We were sick of the border of little yellow duckies and pacifiers that the previous owner had so carefully stenciled on the wall. Clarice and I picked out the paint. We got all the supplies. I set aside the Monday after Christmas to begin. She went off to work. Alone at home I dutifully set to my task. Preparation was a daunting job. Our little music room is full of music, music, more music, and a Steinway grand piano.

I planned to spend all morning in prep, then the afternoon and Tuesday morning painting. I allowed time for meditation. Took a walk. Rode the stationary bike. Ate a decent breakfast. Yet when I started setting up the painting equipment, the all-too-familiar signs of panic jumped around the walls of my gut. I slowed down, practiced deep breathing. The demons clawed at me. I tried to keep working. Gargantuan belches and hiccups began wracking me. I felt like my body would turn inside out. I started hyperventilating. I occasionally involuntarily yelled out to the empty house. I felt like I had to stop, collect myself, and see if I could resume after lunch.

The phone rang. *Oh, no. What if I lose control when I answer?* I took a couple of deep breaths, closed my eyes, and picked up the receiver. I made myself answer in my "professional voice": "Hello. Carroll Stegall." I couldn't believe it. My voice sounded perfectly normal. The caller wanted Clarice for some business with the American Guild of Organists. I was able to answer her question. We chatted for a moment, then completed the conversation. When I hung up, I felt calm. I went back to work, finding myself singing as I worked.

That one unexpected human contact with a person I did not know was the key. It broke the pall. I worked the rest of the day and into the early evening with energy and good spirits, finishing the painting in time for a late supper with my sweetheart.

We were almost to the Millennium. At 8:30 AM on Thursday, December 30, 1999, the phone rang. I heard a monotone voice. "This is Mary from Dr. Shiller's office. He wanted me to call you . . . (long pause) to let you know . . . (pause) that your bone scan . . . (pause) reads clear."

Relief flooded my body. I immediately called Clarice. We rejoiced together.

[Journal, December 30, 1999] My recent, and constant, healing image:
Jesus stands radiant before me.
Light streams from him.
His light envelops me.
Light courses through my veins.
This light permits no shadow.
Bad cells, trying to hide,
are bathed in the light and made whole.

It is really a visual prayer. I invoke the image of healing light daily, several times a day. When in a meditative mode or driving my car or taking a walk, the Christ of the healing light stands before me. His eyes are focused on my eyes. His power surrounds me.

It's not over. The news of a clear bone scan is a momentary relief. It is an important marker on a road that continues. I do not make the road, but I do determine how I will travel it.

The prayer goes further:

May the light that illumines me,
that heals me, continue its healing.
Shine not only into me but also through me.
May my ego stay out of the way!
May that healing light illuminate someone else's soul.

When I hear Mozart done purely, I am aware of the music more than of the performance. The music shines through the performer, undistorted in its divine glory. That is the closest human connection I can make to the healing light of Christ.

Christ of the healing light, heal this world.

CHAPTER 29

A NEW ROAD

We came to the New Year's Eve of the monumental calendar change of 1999–2000. We were at loose ends. Our children were in Virginia, North Carolina, and across town. The across town son had his own parties to attend. Most people we knew were staying home. I felt the empty nest begin to shred. I was the one who made the startling proposal, "Let's go down to the Circle." Monument Circle is the hub around which Indianapolis rotates. I knew the crowds would be oppressive. Traffic would be impossible. Noise would be unbearable. But we had to *do something*. After all, millennia don't come around every year.

Until next year.

I had been a holdout for the *true* Millennium of 2001. Yet, if we are counting from a true calendar that begins with the birth of Jesus, we had already missed it. Nobody knows for sure, but it blurred past in 1996 or 1997. My son heard that the "real" Millennium was 1998. Why? Three times 666 equals 1998 (read the Book of Revelation for that one). Then again, it all becomes irrelevant if we use the Hebrew calendar.

I just wanted it to be over so I would not have to hear "Y2K" again. Roger, our realtor friend, said that he was just going to go to bed on New Year's Eve. He wanted to be asleep when the end of the world came.

After dithering for weeks, we decided to go to our own church for a silent New Year's Eve communion. By then, surrounded by meditation and snuggled with my girlfriend, I felt that going downtown was almost a sacrilege.

Clarice said, "Let's just head up Michigan Road to Eighty-Sixth Street and see what we can find." We figured most restaurants would be packed. If so, we could just go home, fix popcorn, and watch *White Christmas*.

As we turned east from Michigan Road onto Eighty-Sixth Street, I looked over to the left and saw, in a strip mall, a Japanese restaurant I had never seen before. The neon sign read, "Daruma."

"Let's give it a try. It doesn't look too crowded." I swung my little maroon Honda Civic around the traffic island and pulled into the parking lot. We could see through the door that no mobs of people were standing in the lobby. We entered and were greeted by a kimono-clad Japanese lady who shuffled up to us in the time-honored manner.

"Please to take off your shoes." She then led us up three steps to the dining area, where tables were placed at kneeling level. It turned out to be an illusion: The tables were set in wells in the floor, so we could sit on the cushions on the floor and still stretch our legs under the table.

The menu told us the tradition of Daruma. It is built around the Japanese New Year. Legend says that the founder of Zen Buddhism sat in a cave, in lotus position, for seven years, until his arms and legs atrophied and fell off. Thus arose the tradition of the Daruma doll. It is pear-shaped, with no arms or legs. When one receives a Daruma doll, the doll has no eyes. One makes their fondest wish and paints on one eye. When the wish is granted, one paints on the other eye.

The Daruma doll is balanced so that you can tip it over, roll it, even throw it, and it will always right itself—the ancient ancestor to the Weeble. The blessing of the Daruma doll for New Year's is "may you always find your balance, no matter how life treats you."

A week later our Stephen Ministry group met. I shared with them the news of my renewed cancer treatments. Amee is a gentle woman, full of empathy. "How do the treatments make you feel?"

Wanting to keep a light tone, I answered, "Well I might go 'weirding out' on you sometime."

Amee looked up through her eyelashes in the disarming, doe-eyed way she has—probably the same look she used to snare her husband some twenty-five years earlier. "Will we know the difference?"

Within a couple of weeks, it was exam time at school. Students never realize that the teachers themselves experience stress. Just like college music majors, all the students in the music magnet take private music lessons. At the end of each semester, they have to present a "jury," a performance exam before the faculty. As a private voice teacher, I, as well as my students, am under judgment. Each voice student must have three songs prepared to sing from memory. That comes out to nearly ninety different songs. Have I assigned appropriate songs? Have I adequately prepared the students? Are they making acceptable progress? As the jury day progressed, the stress level intensified. We scrambled to finish exams so the students could get to their next classes. Students scrambled to get themselves ready to present their trembling talent. In-between conversations became very loud.

Traumatic performances required interrupting our straight-jacket schedule to comfort, calm, and chastise students.

By mid-afternoon I felt like jumping up on my chair, screaming, and throwing things. My stomach ached. My hands shook. Then I wanted to withdraw into a dark place where no one could find me. The Christ of the transforming light did not appear.

On Sunday morning Amee said, "Something's wrong. You've lost your sparkle." By Monday my spirits were brighter. At Bible study that evening, I told Amee that I had planned to put glitter on my eyes to revive the sparkle, but Clarice did not have any for me to borrow.

The performing arts magnet program is housed in, and encounters all the distractions of, an inner city public high school. "Hall sweeps" round up tardy students and herd them into in-school suspension. Drugs, alcohol, knives, and guns turn up in backpacks. In one week, classes were interrupted by four bomb threats.

One day in January, a student threatened me. I had heard a ruckus in the hallway just outside my room. A girl was getting up from the floor. Two boys were running down the stairs. They were all laughing. As the boys stopped on the stairs to yell up at the girl, I told them to get to class.

One of the boys continued yelling. It took me a few seconds to realize he was now yelling at me. "That's the rudest thing a person can do! Stand there and stare at me! Makes me want to rip off this handrail and hit you across the head with it!"

The three of them then ran downstairs. I turned back into my room and looked in the mirror. *God! I look old! What am I doing here? Is this what I have spent a lifetime preparing for?*

Many mornings I would wake up with a passage from Gian-Carlo Menotti's opera *The Medium* churning through my brain: "O God, forgive my sins, I'm sick and old."[49] The musical phrase would cycle over and over. Even consciously singing another song would not drown it out.

A few days later, a new student came into the performing arts program. He lived, for reasons to which we were not privy, in a group home. He was neat. Clean-cut. Good musical ear. Basic voice okay. Very earnest. I asked, "What attracted you to this program?"

His answer was clear, soft-spoken but unambivalent: "People keep putting me down, telling me I can't do anything. I want to find something I can do really well."

Later that same day, I sought out a senior girl who had missed her lesson earlier in the week. I knew she was going to perform at the school music association solo contest that weekend. "Nikki, come in and let's go over your contest piece."

She slouched into my room, gazing at the floor. I had worked with her for over three years. I knew she had health problems. I also knew her to be exceptionally conscientious. She not only had made up all work missed due to being in the hospital, but was preparing for early graduation. Beautiful and poised, she had been offered the prospect of a recording contract with a rhythm and blues label.

She sang her contest song. It was letter perfect, but totally lacking in energy. Her voice was weak and fuzzy. She sat down.

"What is it, Nikki?"

"I'm pregnant, and I have herpes."

She kept taking a piece of paper out of her pocket, unfolding it, looking at it, refolding it, putting it away. Finally she handed the paper to me. It was a sonogram image. "I had a sonogram this morning. I saw his heart beating. This is a real child. I can't kill my child. I can't bring him into the world knowing he might be deformed. I'm not ready to raise a child. The father is not going to be any help. I can't carry this child and give him up to someone else.

"If my parents find out I'm pregnant, they will kick me out of the house. I have plans for college and a career. My friends are turning against me. They're like: 'I thought you were different. You were an example to us. Now you're just like the rest of us.'"

We spent the next two class periods talking over her fears. She had carefully thought through all the options she knew. All came up as dead ends. I listened, asked questions. I did not ask the obvious. She had already been hit with, "You've done wrong." She had enough guilt to pass around to several others and still have plenty left over. I felt helpless.

That night I presented her dilemma to our Stephen Ministry group. I kept her identity confidential. Several persons had suggestions of places she could turn for help. One even offered to let the girl come live in her home. The next day I took a card to Nikki. I wrote down for her what I had garnered the previous evening. Her face lit up. I could see a weight lifting off her shoulders. "You did all this for me?"

A few days later, I came upon one of my senior students in my room, practicing the piano. For three years he had shown such arrogance, stubbornness, and laziness that I had threatened not to continue teaching him. But toward the end of his junior year, I began to see some change. He is so talented, I had written to his parents, that if he ever actually worked on his music, he could blow the competition off the stage. Now he was doing just that. We chatted for a few minutes. Then he offered: "Dr. Stegall, I want to give you a copy of my portfolio tape. I think you will see that I've made a lot of progress since my freshman year. Despite all my stubbornness, you have helped me a lot." We exchanged a bear hug, and then he went on to his next class.

After he left I thought of another super talent who had graduated three years earlier. Working with him had been hard. He could learn music easily and sound good enough to send the girls into a swoon. That was enough for him.

I fought, struggled, sometimes yelled, to show him a fuller picture of his possibilities. I had known this young man since he was in fourth grade. He had been my son's roommate on trips with the Indianapolis Children's Choir. I had sung in opera chorus with his grandfather. His grandparents were his primary musical supporters. His mom was his disciplinarian. His dad had been largely absent from his life.

"Robert, I love you like a son. So I feel I have a right to chastise you like a father." Maybe I didn't have that right, but I claimed it anyway.

One May morning, during the week Robert was to graduate, he finished his voice lesson, left my room, got partway down the hall, turned around, and came back.

"I'm turning eighteen next month. You know, when you are eighteen, you have the right to change your name. I think I will change my name to Stegall. Richard Carroll Stegall Atkins." Then he sauntered back out, leaving me to pick up my jaw from the floor.[50]

Maybe this is why I am here.

CHAPTER 30

DO WE WANT THIS KIND OF TOGETHERNESS?

On a Sunday evening in February, Clarice and I had a candlelight dinner of grilled cheese sandwiches, chips, pickles, and wine. As we finished dinner, she took my hand and borrowed a line from the old Carol Burnett show: "Are you sitting down, Margaret?"

I checked my chair. "You want me on the floor already?"

"I had a mammogram this week that showed a new growth in my right breast." Her doctor had done a sonogram, and then ordered a needle biopsy. She would get the results the next Wednesday. She already had an appointment with a surgeon.

"You've had all that done and didn't tell me sooner?"

"I didn't tell you right away because I wanted to make sure you were emotionally stable enough to handle the news." That announcement faced me with one of my fears—that I would be inadequate in dealing with her concerns.

The next day she saw her own doctor. He reassured her regarding her biopsy and upcoming exploratory surgery. He indicated that usually they don't amount to anything. Clarice's spirits were positive. Her humor flashed. She showed strength that I could only hope to find a shred of.

We started Valentine's Day with a visit to the breast surgeon. Dr. Tom Schmidt showed clarity, directness, tact, and compassion. He explained that the needle biopsy had indicated some atypical cells. *Atypical* did not mean that the cells were cancerous.

For years Clarice has been conscientious about doing regular self-examinations and having an annual mammogram. The latest mammogram was the first to show anything unusual, so she was ahead of the game.

He needed to do a lumpectomy for a more complete biopsy. He explained that Dr. Harper of the Breast Center would use a sonogram to locate the precise spot for him to excise. Dr. Harper would insert a wire into Clarice's breast, pinpointing the spot. Then I would take Clarice, wire and all, to Women's Hospital, several blocks away, for the surgery. The whole procedure would start at 7:00 AM and be finished by late morning. She could go home by early afternoon and be back to work the next day.

Then the lab would biopsy the questionable tissue. "A well-differentiated carcinoma is a possibility."

I asked, "Dr. Schmidt, will you please explain the term *well-differentiated?* I thought I knew, but now I realize I am unclear."

He explained. "Differentiating relates to cell pattern, rather than size. Level 1 represents an even pattern. Level 3 represents a chaotic pattern."

While he was talking, I had been observing a little wad of tissue stuck to his neck. When he stepped out of the room, I whispered to Clarice, "Does it give you confidence in your surgeon that he cut himself shaving?"

That evening we treated ourselves to the dinner gift certificate the choir had given us for Christmas. We indulged in a sumptuous Valentine's Day Italian dinner at one of the finer restaurants in the Circle Center Mall downtown.

CHAPTER 31

EZEKIEL AND THE RIVER OF LIFE

Merle was in a bind. The pastor was to be away the last Sunday in February. Merle's task was to find a guest preacher. I was in the church office the Wednesday morning Merle stormed in, grousing about being turned down again. I had been feeling really good that morning, singing as I made my usual preparations for choir rehearsal. I turned to him, and said, "I'll do it."

He laughed.

I felt like I had been kicked in the stomach. My emotions fell over an invisible precipice. Initially I tried to cover up, but already the depression was swallowing me. I told Merle, as calmly as I could, what his response had triggered. He reeled backward, then went on the offensive. "Well, if you are going to act that way . . ." He walked away.

I was near tears. This was one of many times when a feather could push me over. After a few minutes, he returned and apologized for being insensitive.

A couple of hours later, he came back, having been turned down by yet another minister. "Are you still interested? I know you as a musician and storyteller. I never thought of you as a regular public speaker." He stammered. "I'm sorry. It never occurred to me."

I'm not that proud. I jumped at the chance.

I set to work. The folklore study I had worked on several years before provided most of the material. The theme traced river imagery as symbols of major life transitions. Starting with Ezekiel, chapter 47, the vision of the river flowing from the temple, it pointed to parallels with a homely Southern folktale I call "Grandpa and the Bullfrogs." Sorry, I can't write it down. You have to hear it and see it.

Using biblical and folklore references, the sermon moved through my own spiritual journey toward the future of our local congregation. I was to preside over the entire worship hour. For the children's time, I used the folktale that served as the basis for the sermon. Clarice got into the act, accompanying on the piano as we wove several songs into the sermon presentation. Because our organ and choir are in the balcony, we usually see just the tops of people's heads, giving us a particular perspective on bald spots and comb-overs. On this Sunday, though, I could look people in the eye. I could feel them come with me into what, by any accounts, was an unusual worship experience. The theme of rivers and life transitions allowed me to reveal some personal events that our current congregation did not know:

Four times I have crossed over the Mississippi River in moves that represented major life changes. Clarice and I, married scarcely one year, left the not-so-hallowed halls of academic life and the capital of the Confederacy to cross over the Mississippi into Iowa. There we found a great university in a cosmopolitan city that was plopped in the middle of cornfields. Through that city ran the Iowa River.

Five years later, with a fresh degree, two new children, and a beagle in tow, we crossed back over the Mississippi to seek academic grandeur on the banks of the Ohio. Soon we found ourselves perched on top of the Blue Ridge Mountains, ten miles from the headwaters and one hundred yards from the banks of the New River. Actually, our house was in the New River when the hundred-year flood came.

Back across the Mississippi to Southwest Oklahoma, lured by promises of prestige, promotion, and prosperity. Instead we descended into our personal, predestined six years of purgatory. What passed for rivers were mainly dried up creek beds.

Yet along the way, I found my soul.

Thoroughly purged of all pretensions of finding the meaning of life in academia, we once again crossed the Mississippi to come to the Heartland, Clarice's home state, and the Circle City thirteen years ago. I now teach on the banks of the White River.

Our lives keep changing. Children out of school and on their own. Family deaths, marriages, births. Three dogs replaced by two foster cats. A five-year quest[51] to master cancer while trying to accept its place in my life.

Several years ago I experienced a vivid, lucid dream: I found a river. It was heavily polluted. Through great effort, and after successive failures, I reached the headwaters. I saw pure water bubbling from a rock. Then I followed the river back downstream. The river widened, becoming full of commerce and pollution. Now I was in a small rowboat. I was rowing, but someone else was handling the tiller. Whenever the little boat turned, the water became pure. I looked back and saw that the person at the tiller was Jesus.

With Clarice accompanying on the piano, I closed the sermon by singing Aaron Copland's setting of "At the River," with its refrain so familiar to millions:

> Yes, we'll gather by the river,
> the beautiful, the beautiful river,
> gather with the saints by the river
> that flows by the throne of God.[52]

The lights in people's eyes told me. They traveled with me every step. Afterward an octogenarian grasped my hand. "I wanted to put my hands together and clap, but it's just not . . . not . . ."

"Decent and in order?" I finished his sentence.

"You got it!" He laughed with me.

Another friend said, "I wanted to stand up and tell everybody how fortunate we are to have Clarice and Carroll in our church." As gratified as I felt with those and similar responses, I really wanted the emphasis to be on the message, not the messenger.

The whole process was building toward another crash. On Monday I had early voice lessons to teach at Broad Ripple. I also had to get a new PSA test done. The triple whammy of Monday, a letdown from a high, and PSA anxiety, not to mention worry about Clarice's condition, split me into three parts that engaged in an out-loud dialogue. It was not just my imagination, and it was not just thoughts.

The Emotional Self cried out, "**O God, help me!**"

The Rational Self answered, *"What is it? Are you afraid?"*

"**God, I'm so scared!**"

"What are you afraid of?"

"**I don't know.**" Tears were flowing. Throat was tight. Voice was broken.

"You are starting to calm down. Don't go away. Don't hide it. Tell me what you are afraid of." The voice was calm, reassuring.

"**Dying.**"

"Dying." The Rational Self repeated, the voice reflective. The throat was not tight. No tears. *"Even though you have said for forty years that you were not afraid of death."*

"**It's—pain—dependence. It's—not knowing! It's—what if the PSA shoots up again? What if treatments are no longer any good? What if everything I believe, everything I have been taught is a lie? All the stuff about death being a transition to a new and better life—*What if it is a lie?*"**

The Rational Self was silent.

The whole time a spectator, a third part of me, was quietly observing.

Had anyone heard my dialogue between the rational voice and the emotional voice, they would have been ready to commit me. They were two distinct voices. One was calm, rational, well modulated. The other was choked with sobs, short of breath, wailing. But they both came out of my mouth and my soul.

I called school. *If I'm late, I'm late.* I pulled into a meditative mode, then slept.

This internal confrontation had been many years in the making. Much of my life has been a spiritual search. Among my earliest memories are questions of morals or spirit. Although as a child, I had heard many sermons about how terrible hell was, I never really believed that the sermons applied to me. I was "saved," baptized by believer baptism when I was six years old.

My only childhood questioning came when Daddy took us into Winston-Salem to swim at Reynolds Park. I was in third grade. As I jumped into the pool in my old wool bathing suit, I thought, *If heaven doesn't have swimming pools, I'm not sure I want to go there.*

The next year I received, much as had the boy Samuel, a midnight "call," which my child mind interpreted as my destiny to be a minister. I would gradually come to realize that music, not pastoring, was my passion. I saw Daddy praying with the sick, comforting the bereaved, bailing out drunks. Those duties terrified me. When I confided my fears to Mother, she said, "The Lord will give you strength." End of discussion.

I entered Wake Forest College[53] in 1959. I never considered another college. At that time it was the only four-year co-ed Baptist college in North Carolina. I registered as a preministerial student, intending to major in religion, philosophy, or psychology. During my freshman year, I realized that, for nearly ten years, every time I thought about pastoring, a voice had whispered, *I hope I get a small church where I can direct the choir.* Though I had begun questioning the literal nature of the Bible in high school, a germ of belief was always there. My freshman Old Testament professor at Wake Forest was Dan O. Via, who was later to enter the front ranks of biblical scholars with his study of the parables of Jesus. Dan Via introduced me to the idea of progressive revelation, the concept that through the centuries, people of faith discover new things about God. "The revelation may be perfect, but the receiver is imperfect," he intoned to his soporific freshman class. That concept touched a chord with me.

The next significant faith event still sounds strange to my ears, even after the passage of four decades. The summer after I graduated from high school, my parents moved to another town to take jobs teaching school. Daddy soon became interim pastor at a little mission. His charge was to prepare it to become chartered as a church. When I had a rare weekend at home, the only thing to do was to go to church with my parents. I dreaded going back into the fundamentalist environment of which I was trying to cleanse myself. My parents were conservative evangelicals, not capital-F Fundamentalists, although a number of their church folk were. I warned Mother not to volunteer me to sing. I silently hoped nobody would ask me to pray.

The preacher that Sunday was the closest facsimile to an old-fashioned hellfire-and-brimstone preacher that I had heard since I was a young boy. His manner was arrogant. His voice was bombastic. His message was repulsive. He used all the classic evangelistic tricks in his invitation call. He knew how to milk guilt and fear.

My tender attempts at academic objectivity were no match. Against my will I was pulled onto my feet and down to the altar. The evangelist raised his arms in triumphal praise, then leaned over and placed his hands on my head. I murmured that I wanted to rededicate my life.

Sitting in the back seat of Daddy's car on the way back to their house, I marveled. I told my parents, "This preacher represents everything I am trying to free myself of. Yet the spirit I felt was real. I now know that God is with me."

In a late-night dormitory bull session a few weeks later, the discussion turned to life and death, faith and doubt. A suite mate whirled around to me. "Stegall, do you believe in heaven?"

Without thinking it through, I heard myself saying: "I really don't know. What I do know is that my relationship with God is a personal one. Whatever he has in store after I die is okay by me."

Faith questions were not settled, however. I still sometimes doubted God's existence. Each new question posed a new struggle. My senior year, in the spring of 1963, I had occasion to speak in a debate at the North Carolina Baptist State Convention, in Raleigh. At issue was alleged "worldliness and non-Baptist teaching" at Wake Forest.

Prodded by my girlfriend, I took an open mike and said, in part: "Academic study and questioning of beliefs have not weakened my faith. Rather, they have strengthened it. If my faith cannot stand criticism, my faith cannot stand."

The next day Dan Via stopped me on campus and thanked me for my courage.

"Thank you, Dr. Via, but I did not think I was courageous. I was just mad!"

Even though I still went through periods of being what Marcus Borg calls "a closet agnostic,"[54] I was always active in church. Public worship was important to me. I have always believed that we are, in some fashion, eternal.

I remained skeptical about prayer, wondering if it was not just another means of giving ourselves a pep talk. In a covenant group in the late 1970s, our leader asked each of us to tell how prayer had affected our lives. When it came my turn, I responded: "I confess that I have not believed in, or practiced, prayer in the fullest sense of the word. But for the first time in my life, I now want to."

All the time I longed to be a mystic. I came to realize that the hymn "Spirit of God, Descend upon My Heart" did not speak to my craving. One stanza claims:

> I ask no dream, no prophet ecstasies,
> No sudden rending of the veil of clay,
> No angel visitant, no opening skies,
> But take the dimness of my soul away.[55]

What this hymn denies is exactly what I sought. I wanted dreams. I wanted ecstasies. I wanted angels. I wanted signs to validate my beliefs. Along the way I did experience signs. Some I accepted; others I ignored, rejected, or more often, just plain did not recognize.

Another stanza of that same hymn goes further in denying what my soul needed, when it pleads for strength "to check the rising doubt, the rebel sigh." I have believed for decades that doubt and rebellion are essential elements of growing faith.

But that primal scream of despair had kept silent.

Until now.

The Emotional Self had to be goaded by the Rational Self to release itself from its half-century prison. Once released, it found some peace.

Back in real time, I awoke an hour later refreshed and ready to face the day, beginning with the trek to the hospital lab to get my PSA blood draw.

Our regular Bible study group met that evening. We rotated meeting in homes. On the way to the meeting, I listened as Clarice told me about a bizarre day she had experienced at her office. Then I told Clarice about my experience of that morning. As I talked, I tried to stay composed. I tried to fight back tears. Both efforts failed. We were still talking about it as we neared our destination. She volunteered to whip out her cell phone and tell our hosts that we could not come.

"No. I need to go. I want to see my friends."

Our hosts greeted us, as did their yippy little terrier. Their home is an inviting mix of modern architecture and antique furnishings. Encouraged by the warmth of the surroundings and their easy hospitality, I managed to put on my "party face" and greet everyone as if all were normal. They gave Clarice and me lots of affirmations about the worship of the previous day.

Among the study group were Amee and Sven, as well as two other members of the Stephen Ministry, one of whom was also a choir member. Sven and another one of the men kept repeating the refrain to the folktale I had told the children, then cackling like kids themselves. My tension began to release.

However, as we got into the meat of the discussion about the Samaritan woman at the well, I could feel the signs of panic beginning to arise. *I can't sit here much longer.* I got up, went to the bathroom, came back, and lay down on the floor. "I'm still with you. I just need to stretch out."

"Oh. Is your back bothering you?"

"No. I'm just very worn out."

I closed my eyes and tried to visualize a peaceful scene while still participating in the discussion. In a minute I felt something wet on my face. It was the terrier, Ginger, equal parts ears, fur, and tongue. She lay down in the crook of my arm where she could look up and study my face.

Our host tried to shoo the dog away.

Clarice said: "It's okay. Our cats do that all the time."

"But she never does this. Even when we are lying on the floor."

Occasionally Ginger would give me a slurp or nuzzle my neck. But mainly she just lay there and let me ruffle her fur. *So she never behaves like this, huh? She knows something the humans don't. They think I have a bad back. She knows I have a hurting heart.* Ginger was my therapist.

Depression continued to gnaw at me much of the week, though most of the time I was able to override it and continue what I had to do. At our Stephen Ministry meeting on Thursday evening, I reported that I was to get my PSA results the next day. "If the reading is down by a large margin, I will ask not to take the next treatment, because it has done its job. If it is up significantly, I likely will not take the treatment, because it will show that it's no longer effective."

I must have sounded more discouraged than I intended, for my colleagues started asking me questions designed to buoy me up. I asked Amee to stay after the meeting. I told her about the strange internal conversation of Monday, and leveled with her about my fight with panic during the Bible study. We also talked about Clarice's upcoming breast surgery. Amee had run the whole breast cancer gamut, so she had some encouraging insights for me.

Clarice had been at church that same evening for another meeting. After her meeting she breezed through to say good-bye before she headed home. Amee and I continued talking for more than an hour. She seemed to have something on her mind, something that she hesitated to bring up.

Finally, she ventured, "Is it okay with Clarice for us to talk like this?"

"Of course. I can't dump on her all the time."

"I don't know . . . I get a funny feeling. . . ."

Then I caught her drift. I shook my head and grinned. "I have seen Clarice when she felt like her territory was being invaded. Believe me, this ain't it!"

When I got home, I related to Clarice my talk with Amee, and Amee's concern. Her reply was essential Clarice. "I'm glad you have a friend you can talk to. If I *were* to get jealous, everybody better watch out!" She did not have to remind me of the times that bright young students had come to see their voice teacher as more than a teacher. My wife's wrath can turn steel into cinders.

By Friday afternoon, when I had not heard from the doctor about the latest PSA, I decided it was high time to find out. Between classes I went to the one general-access phone in the building, which was in the teacher's lounge. The phone was in use, with another person waiting. I hated to use my cell phone because we don't have free minutes, and I didn't want to spend a week's income plowing through voice-mail recordings.

But I did it anyway.

"You have reached Urology Associates. If you know the extension you want, dial it now. For appointments, press *one*. For the nurse, press *two*. To find out if you are going to die, press *three*." That's what I heard anyway.

I pressed *three*.

"This is Bonnie. How may I help you?"

"I want to get my PSA results."

"What's your Social?"

I rattled off the numbers, as familiar as my own name.

"Just a moment."

My cell phone beeped the lapsing minutes as I listened to elevator music.

"Mr. Stegall? Your file is on Dr. Shiller's desk. I can't give you the results until he has had time to study them."

Not a good sign.

I gave her Clarice's number. Phoning me at school is futile. And I didn't want my cell phone going off in the middle of a lesson.

After school I stopped in at Clarice's office. "Have you heard from Dr. Shiller?"

"Yes."

"Do you have the results?"

"Yes."

I looked at her hard, over my glasses. "Do I need to sit down?"

"Yes."

I sat down. "Okay. What is it?" The December reading had been 70.97. Her answer told me to prepare for a rise. I braced myself for it to be up to, maybe, 90.0.

Clarice looked me in the eye. "Two oh two."

I gave her my best you-gotta-be-kidding grin. "Isn't there a period in there somewhere? Twenty point two?"

"No."

"Two point oh two?"

"No."

"What about point two oh two?"

"No. There is no period."

"Two hundred and two." I sank down in the chair. "Oh, my God!"

I knew she hated telling me. I had put on the wise-guy act to shield us both. My wife should not have to be the one to break news like that. The pros are supposed to do it. But she *was* a pro. Calm. Clear. Direct. Compassionate. Dr. Shiller had told her that he would not give me the shot scheduled for that week. Instead, I must see Dr. Logan, the oncologist, as soon as possible. He would outline the next treatment scenario.

It had finally happened. The hormones had become ineffective.

Clarice came around from her desk and held me in a long embrace. We then turned to practical matters. The test results pushed aside all the confusion. For four years I had been caught in a thicket. Treatments could push the boundaries of the thicket back a little. But I was always surrounded. There was no path through the thicket. Now we had a path. Not of our choosing, but we had a path.

"I want you to go with me when I see Dr. Logan. He will be giving out a lot of information. I hate to pull you out right after your own surgery, but I'll need an extra head to absorb it all."

Knowing how fuzzy I can get on details, she agreed. I made an appointment for the following Thursday, two days after her surgery.

We turned our attention to Clarice's lumpectomy. I arranged for my Tuesday morning women's chorus to hold sectional rehearsals on their own so I could stay with Clarice. She remained bright, upbeat, and humorous about it. Yet at 6:30 Tuesday morning, on the way to the Breast Center, she said: "I'm more apprehensive about this procedure than I was about my hysterectomy. I'm not sure why. Maybe because it is external instead of internal."

"Also," I responded, "when you had the hysterectomy, you knew that the surgery was all there was to it. It was over. With this one, we don't know what the results will be. But remember: We are in it together!"

She came through the surgery groggy but in good spirits. She worked a half day the next day, and directed our choir in an ecumenical Ash Wednesday service. My biggest test was helping her change the dressing. To my surprise, I didn't throw up or even flinch.

On Friday we got the word. The biopsy was clear. No evidence of cancer. I told her that if I had needed to write a love song about "My Lopsided Lover," I would have done so with gratitude that I still had her.

CHAPTER 32

HOW DO YOU FIRE
AT AN INVISIBLE ENEMY?

We sat in a tiny waiting room. The TV was blasting out the soaps. To override the TV, conversations were loud. I looked at the glass door and read the backside of the etched lettering: Oncology and Hematology. I never really believed I would be here. As I filled out my case history, my stomach began to tighten. It was Thursday. We had not yet gotten Clarice's results.

The nurse called me in. "And how are we doing today?"

"It may be my apprehension, but it seems awfully noisy out there."

"Well, Hon, we'll try to do something about that." She put her hand on my shoulder as I stepped onto the scale. She went out and turned the TV volume off.

A few minutes later, she called Clarice and me back to the consultation room, where we met with Dr. Logan. He was just like I remembered him from our first meeting three years earlier. Tall, with a runner's lean body, he is a hot-wired bundle of energy. I handed him a copy of a graph I had been keeping. It charted all treatments and PSA readings since 1994. I felt pleased that he could read my entire case history from the graph.

He used his dry-erase board to write down for us what he was saying. Clarice and I both whipped out our notepads and wrote furiously.

"You have a rise in PSA, but no symptoms. It appears that the hormones have run their course. I suggest that you take another one-month shot as a check. You don't need to bother with the Casodex. Just the Lupron. There is a 95 percent chance that the PSA will continue rising.

If it does, then we will have clear evidence that the hormones are no longer effective. In clinical trials we require two successive failures to prove the experiment a failure. If the PSA comes back down, then we can treat the current rise as an aberration and continue on the hormones. However, there is less than a 5 percent chance of that happening. In any case we will have a clearer idea of how to proceed."

My head swirled. I did not even want to consider more hormone treatments. I had actually seen this current rise as a chance to be free of treatments and maybe to feel normal for a while.

Dr. Logan continued. "If the PSA continues to rise and you have no symptoms, then I suggest we do nothing until you get symptoms. The rise in PSA is a precursor to symptoms. We cannot tell you how much time will pass before you experience symptoms. It could be weeks, months, or as much as a year. However, we will usually see symptoms within a year." He went on to explain that a tripled PSA does not indicate tripled cancer activity. There is no direct correlation between the PSA reading and the size of a tumor. "Although a higher reading does show greater abnormal activity, it is not a one-to-one relationship." PSA readings may sometimes run as high as twenty to thirty thousand.

Symptoms would not show up until the cancer became localized. He reinforced what I had heard so many times before. It would likely show up in the bones, lymph nodes, or lungs.

"In those cases we can try spot radiation, mild chemo, or steroids such as prednisone. We can also inject a radioactive isotope into the blood to strengthen the bones. Aredia is a substance that has been FDA approved for breast cancer and multiple myeloma, when they spread to the bones. Aredia is awaiting FDA approval for prostate cancer in the bones. It is for well-defined bone spots. It would retard the cancer from eating into the bones.

"It will not halt the cancer, just give the bones a stronger barrier. It will be like turning balsa wood into oak. We have no data saying whether presymptom treatment will prolong life."

He was participating in a study that addressed that question, but the data were not all in. The results would not be known for several years.

They would have to wait for subjects to die.

He also offered us the option of having further tests, such as a CT scan, a chest X ray, and another bone scan. But, he added, even if they find something, he did not see any point in treating until it bothered me.

"So, finding a hot spot would be mainly academic information at this point?"

"Exactly."

I told him that I was writing a journal about my experience and that I had a publisher interested. "May I quote you? May I use your name?"

"Sure. I have confidence that everything I have told you will hold up anywhere in the world. And in the movie, I want to be played by Kevin Costner!"

❈

Daughter Joi, son-in-law Joe, and granddaughter Emily were to spend a December weekend with us. On Saturday morning I stayed home while Clarice went to church for her regular organ practice. I did some house-cleaning as I waited for Joi's family. I also waited for a service person to come and reprogram our home alarm system. He came mid-morning and spent an hour, testing the alarm every few minutes. The alarm is unnerving anytime. It is designed to scare the juice out of burglars. Having it go off at random was the same as being stuck like a voodoo doll. You never knew when it would hit. You just knew it would. And you knew it would be painful.

While he was still working on the alarm system, the kids arrived. We caught up on each other's lives, holding our ears and trying to shout over the recurring alarm. As much as I dote on Emily, as much as I love Joi and Joe, by early Saturday afternoon, I felt the room closing in on me. I pulled myself out of the activity and tried to compose myself. Clarice came back to the bedroom and found me shaking and hyperventilating. She gently rubbed my arms and shoulders, and brought me a dose of Klonopin, calming me enough so that I could sleep.

When I awoke from my nap, Clarice told me that they were talking about getting our family and Joe's family together to go out for dinner. I tried to be a good sport, but felt like I could not cope with such an outing. I said, "Okay, but I don't want any medical talk." Joe's dad would give me his own prostate case update in excruciating detail. His mom would pepper me with advice.

Then we looked out and saw snow falling. It kept coming, finally reaching more than eight inches. *Thank you, God! We don't have to go out!* Joi and Clarice went to the grocery store. Jeremy came over. He and Joi cooked up a fabulous steak dinner, with two kinds of wine, cooked onions, mixed vegetables, and wild rice. Clarice and I cleaned up. We had a grand evening in our dining room with daughter, son, son-in-law, and granddaughter. I just wished Jon were there.

On Monday Clarice e-mailed Jon:

> We saw Dad's oncologist on Thursday. . . . Because Dad has no symptoms, there is no reason to try to do anything until he does. In the meantime, Dad was due for a Lupron shot that same day, which he had cancelled because the urologist said the hormone therapy obviously wasn't working. The oncologist, however, encouraged him to have one more shot (a one-month dose instead of three-month) and get another reading. . . . Dad was reluctant to get another shot, as the treatment makes him feel yucky. However, the doctor said it is probably the supplemental pill that makes him feel bad, and to just leave it off, because it has minimal effectiveness anyway. So next week Dad will get a one-month shot and see what happens. He has lots of days of fragile emotional state, which is frustrating to him and scary to me.
>
> I have my post-op exam a week from today. I itch, so I guess I'm healing!
>
> I was able to pull Emily into a chair with me, but couldn't lift her from the floor. What a character she is! Love, Mom

The earliest date Dr. Shiller's office could schedule me for a consultation and a Lupron shot was the following Tuesday, 8:30 AM. *I have already missed one rehearsal with my women's chorus due to Clarice's lumpectomy. Now I have to be late for another. The ladies will start thinking I'm a slacker!* When I found out that they had said a special prayer for Clarice on the day of her surgery, I knew they would be forgiving.

When I explained to the chorus that I might be a little late for the next rehearsal, one of them asked if I had to get an IV.

"No. It's a shot. I just have to moon a nurse for ten seconds."

As the ensuing uproar calmed down, a sixty-five-year-old alto shouted over the laughter, "Oh, well, 'parts is parts'!" They are so delicate, these grandmothers.

CHAPTER 33

LOVE YOUR ENEMY

March 20, 2000. The first day of spring. Skies overcast, with intermittent rain. Warm, except when gusts of damp air hit you. It did not matter. I felt good. My life had spring in it. When I got to school, one of the first greetings came from a tall, beautiful, blond student: "Happy first day of spring, Dr. Stegall!"

"And a happy first day of spring to you, Bev!"

That greeting warmed me for more than the obvious reasons. The previous year, this young woman had been dragged through hell due to events stemming from the murder of a close friend. She was always something of a loner, but she had become increasingly withdrawn, physically separating herself from other students in the classroom.

Bev was bright and talented, but she lived in fear and isolation.

Now we were observing a transformation. She re-engaged in extracurriculars. She and friends would run up to each other for hugs and loud greetings. Her singing began to blossom. I put her in an honors recital. I told her dad that I believed his daughter could learn any music; I did not see any technical limitations. She began to sing with passion.

One morning, when I had found it a major effort to put one foot in front of the other, Bev had come to her voice lesson and, as my revered teacher Herald "Prof" Stark used to say, "Sang the pants off that music."

At the end of her lesson, I said, "You have brightened my morning." She didn't just brush it off. She turned back from the door. "Why? What's wrong?"

I wasn't expecting that. But since she had shown startling candor during her crisis, I decided not to cover up. "I was pretty depressed this morning. You helped bring me out of it."

She seemed incredulous. "What would you have to be depressed about?"

I had opened up as far as I dared to at that moment. "It has to do with some medication I'm taking. But I'm okay now. Have a great weekend."

She skipped across my tiny studio and gave me a hug. "Feel better," she piped, then darted out of the door to her next class.

❀

Back to the first day of spring in the year we number two thousand. In the afternoon I wrote a longhand letter to my across-town child.

> For the first time in a couple of weeks, I feel normal. This is a good time to share some feelings with you. I was just reading something that jumped off the page at me: "I, too, must stand and watch the sufferings of my dear ones; the heartaches, sicknesses, and grief of those I love. And I must let them watch mine, too."[56] I have shielded you from part of myself, not because I really wanted to, but because I did not want to upset you. Mom fills you in on things, but I want you to hear this from me.
>
> After riding in a "safe" zone for around sixteen months, my PSA rose from 3.55 in July to 70.97 in December. We resumed treatments in December. This time, however, the PSA kept rising, to 202.0 in March. Dr. Shiller sent me to Dr. Logan, an oncologist (cancer specialist). Tomorrow I will take one more Lupron (hormone) shot as a double check. Dr. Logan believes, as does Dr. Shiller, that the hormones have lost their effectiveness. This treatment is mainly to verify their suspicions.
>
> No localized cancer has been found. There is no need for further treatments until it does become localized. How do I feel? Apprehensive. Frightened. Relieved that I can be free of the treatments

for a while! Meanwhile I am doing everything I know how to keep healthy through diet, exercise, and meditation. I admit to a craving for chocolate and caffeine!

I know that you do not endorse the Christianity I do. I also know that you are a spiritual person. I suspect that you have a mystical streak, as do I. I must let you know my feelings. I am incomplete otherwise. And you deserve to know.

We do not know when, or whether, symptoms might arise. That is the cause for hope and the cause for concern. I want to be completely honest with you. I also want to tell you—because it can never be said enough—that I love you. I never heard those words from my own father. I want to make sure that you never forget them. Love, Dad

The next day I met with my urologist, Dr. Shiller. He went over the case, confirming Dr. Logan's findings of asymptomatic elevating PSA. He reminded me that it was my choice. It was up to me whether or not to take the Lupron shot. Before proceeding, I had some questions.

"Dr. Logan mentioned using steroids, such as prednisone. Does that work by shrinking tissue?"

"Partly. It can shrink tissue and reduce inflammation. It can make you feel better. It can increase your appetite. In rare cases it can cause hip damage. We don't know for sure whether it will actually delay cancer growth."

"Dr. Logan told me he had seen PSAs up to twenty and thirty thousand. How high can they go without symptoms?"

"I have seen as much as two to three thousand without symptoms. I have also seen metastatic cancers with much lower PSAs."

He gave me a flyer about PC-SPES, an herbal treatment. It had been in use for several years, but not on a widespread basis. The flyer claimed dramatic results in reducing PSA, but there was no clinical evidence that it actually reduced the cancer. Depending on the dosage one chose, it would cost from $400 to $625 per month. Being nonprescription, insurance would not cover it.

I decided to take the Lupron shot. The nurse came in. "Do you have a cheek of choice?" I asked.

"Yep. Left side up."

Fifteen seconds later I was pulling my pants back on. All over.

The next day Clarice pulled more information about PC-SPES off the Internet. We both looked it over. We agreed not to pursue it. Why pay that much money, which we didn't have, for a treatment with no demonstrated disease-reducing properties?

※

I enjoyed nearly a week of feeling normal. No dizziness, depression, nausea, or panic attacks. Full energy. Brisk, invigorating walks. Singing felt good. I was able, as in days of yore, to sing in the range of my highest sopranos.[57]

On Sunday afternoon I started feeling agitated. By Monday morning, full-blown depression hit again. I started crying as I kissed Clarice before she left for work. Tuesday morning I found myself screaming in the privacy of my car as I headed out for work. I wanted to curse myself for submitting to a treatment that all agreed was probably futile.

By the following Sunday evening, some equilibrium returned. It was past time for a call to an old friend. I dialed the familiar number. The voice answered on the second ring. I started in, "God was loafing around heaven with nothing to do, so decided to torment my old friend Arthur."

"Carroll, *mon ami,* how good to hear from you!"

Arthur Smith is the only person in the world I would ever address in such a manner. He is the only one who calls me *"mon ami."* We had taught, laughed, and suffered together in my earlier incarnation as associate professor of music at a southwest Oklahoma university. Arthur is the only person from that phase of my life whom I still call just to chat. We had not talked since Christmas. Much catching up was in order.

Arthur's beloved wife, Helen, had developed Alzheimer's disease at the unjustly young age of fifty-six or so. By the time she was in her early sixties, she often did not recognize her husband. He kept her at home, arranged around-the-clock care for her, and, with the selfless aid of his daughter, managed a reasonably normal professional life as professor of music—teaching theory and composition and creating his own musical compositions. Just as he was gearing up to retire, he was pressed into service as music department chair, because he was the only person on the faculty whom everyone trusted. Fretting over a fractious faculty, teaching, and composing, as well as caring for a sick wife, just about undid him.

During the time we taught together in the early and mid-1980s, he had written two song cycles for Clarice and me. He also had composed a mass for my college choir. Our professional rapport had developed into a warm friendship and then a truly loving relationship.

On this Sunday evening, I informed Arthur of my escalating PSA. I also told him that we believed that the effectiveness of the treatments was wearing thin. He was stunned. "But you had gone for so long with everything seemingly in control. Yet you seem to have a great serenity about it."

"Well, Arthur, I had to give myself a good talking to. Have you ever carried on an out-loud conversation with yourself?"

"Oh, yes. Back when I was taking care of Helen, I would go in the closet, scream, and beat on the walls, then come out and say, 'Now, Arthur, you've got to get control of yourself!'"

If I was going crazy, I had good company.

"As soon as one hears *cancer*, they shut down." The setting: the St. Vincent Marten House in Indianapolis. The date: April 5, 2000. The event: a forum on "Congregational Care of Those in Illness and Crisis." Amee and another colleague joined me in representing the Stephen Ministry program at Saint Andrew. The speaker: Father Bill Hubmann, oncology chaplain at St. Vincent Hospital, in Indianapolis. Father Hubmann was on a panel representing the wide range of chaplaincy services of a hospital that puts mind-body-spirit wellness in the heart of its mission statement. The guest convener for the day was Dr. Peter Steinke. Dr. Steinke used the human organism as the foundation for understanding family and social relationships. Following his keynote address, the panel took over.

Father Hubmann said: "Fighting to stay alive is healthy to a point. But there comes a time to say good-bye."

As he made his presentation, several questions leapt into my mind. I finally got my turn to ask them. "How do you distinguish among passive acquiescence, denial, and acceptance? How do you distinguish between 'I'm gonna fight this thing' and being an activist patient?"

His answer was clarity itself. "Passivity, denial, and fighting are emotional reactions. Acceptance and actively participating in your healing are rational responses." The distinction, then, is between reacting (an emotional, nonrational act) and responding (a rational, thought-through act).

"Is accepting one's death a positive response?"

Another panelist answered, "I can only respond to something I accept."

I continued with a corollary question. "Do you slay the dragon or do you make friends with the dragon?"

"Yes."

When we had a break in the proceedings, I turned to Amee. "When you discovered you had cancer, did any of these words describe your actions: passivity, denial, fighting, acceptance, activist?"

She did not hesitate. "Passive denial. And I did it all with a smile on my face. I pulled the strings so tight around the back of my head that my mask always showed a smile. What a faker I was!"

Her reply intrigued me. I asked her to tell me more.

"I was desperately trying to hold on to the person I used to be. But she was gone, and the only thing left was a chaotic jumble of anxiety that left me sleepless, depressed, and not 'belonging' anywhere. I couldn't trust myself; I was physically uncomfortable with myself. I didn't connect with that person in the mirror.

"I don't remember how or when, but one day God blessed me with a friend—me. I'm getting to know her, and to value the God-given peace that now brings connectedness and more harmony to my life.

"Whoa, Carroll—aren't you glad you asked? Let's get some lunch!"

She confessed that she had never formed words for her struggle until I put the question flat at her. One thing a trusted friend can do is to hold up a mirror, let you see yourself, and assure you that no matter what you see, that friend still totally accepts you.

I reminded Amee that in my first session with Cyndi almost four years earlier, Cyndi had turned the mirror on me. She had confronted my apparent lack of anger. Then she had prayed for me as I faced my death.

Amee is coming to know a new person. She is making friends with the new Amee. That new person arises from her confrontation with death. Death, burial, and resurrection are not a one-time event. It is not only the coward who "dies a thousand deaths."[58] We travel through many deaths, many burials, many resurrections in the course of one lifetime. Yet we carry with us all those former lives. They overlap one another in the complexity of tributaries that merge into streams and rivers.

✳

As the year 2000 progressed, so did my PSA. Still, I thought it was better to have a high asymptomatic PSA than to go through all the bad effects of renewed treatment. I wrote to my doctors:

June 13, 2000. Five years ago today, Dr. Shiller informed me of the diagnosis of a moderately active prostate malignancy. With asymptomatic PSA changing precipitously and erratically, I have decided, after counsel with Dr. Shiller, Dr. Logan, and my family, to discontinue the treatment plan (Lupron and Casodex) I have followed since April 1996. I am grateful that the treatment has been effective for nearly four yours. By conservative estimate, during the time that I have been under treatment, 75 percent of those days, I have experienced some degree of nausea, diarrhea, anxiety, depression, hot flashes, or sudden onslaughts of fatigue. My wife says that I am not much fun when under treatment! When I am not on treatments, all those effects diminish. My energy and sense of well being increase.

In the event that the cancer should become acute enough to create another generation of symptoms, I have some specific requests:

Do not tell me I have X number of months to live. Do not tempt the chance of a self-fulfilling prophecy.

Do not conspire to secrecy. I know that my doctors would not do that anyway. This request goes for everybody—especially family and friends.

Do give me the complete diagnosis.

Do give me the statistical norms.

Do give me and my family full information about possible treatments.

Do acknowledge that my disease is part of my life; and is as unique as I am.

Do respect my belief in the interrelationships among mind, body, and spirit.

Do accept my decisions regarding further treatments.

Do challenge me when you think I am going cockeyed!

I chose to stay off treatments while the PSA fluctuated wildly, reaching a high of 528. I kept checking in with Dr. Adams, who would always ask,

"How do you feel—today?" In the early fall, I answered: "Waiting for the next brick to fall. With an astronomical asymptomatic PSA, I know something will change. I just don't know what, when, where, or how."

Clarice and I determined not to wait around and see what was going to happen. In that period of uncertainty, we decided to grab hold of life and ride. As the fall of 2000 approached, we geared up for our long-planned trip to Austria, Germany, and Italy, focused on the millennial performance of the Oberammergau Passion Play. I had never before taken a vacation while school was in session. As soon as school started, I met each of my private voice students and laid out, in detail, what work each of them was to prepare while I was away.

Our children had given us a set of luggage for Christmas. I needed to allow extra luggage space to haul my medications and supplies, so I could be prepared for my continuing depression, panic attacks, fatigue, nausea, diarrhea, and leaky bladder. Those factors proved to be mere inconveniences in the rich experience that would unfold during the weeks of our trip.

We traveled with people we had already met, several of whom Clarice had worked with. It was a continuing party. For the first week, we kept a home base in Oberperfuss, a little village in the Austrian Alps. Looking at the brochure, I thought, *No way can this place be as charming as the picture.* To my absolute astonishment, it was better than the promo pictures.

The Passion play itself, an all-day event in a huge amphitheater, is worth the price and the wait. It dominates the economy, the labors, the talents, and the spirit of the tiny German village of Oberammergau. *Ammer* is the name of a river. The name *Oberammergau* means "Upper Ammer Valley." There is also an Unterammergau, "Lower Ammer Valley."

During the year of the Passion play production, all village work goes toward it. Village elders hold a ceremony in which they renew the Oath of 1643, dedicating every tenth year exclusively to the service of God through re-enacting the Passion.

Cast members are selected a year ahead of the performances, and are expected to let their lives be infused by the spirit of the characters. That demand must take an awful toll on the high priests Caiaphas and Annas, Roman governor Pilate, King Herod, and the betrayer, Judas Iscariot. Their dedication gets further tests. Performances are five days a week from April to October. During the performances the audience is under a protective shell. The stage is all outdoors. The rationale for this peculiar structure is that the Passion play requires total dedication. Something like a mere summer thunderstorm becomes a witness to that dedication as the performance continues uninterrupted.

They perform without electronic amplification to an audience of five thousand. The role of *Christus* is powerful, commanding. He makes you understand why the Roman and ecclesiastical authorities were afraid of him. No "sweet little Jesus boy." No matter how careful the production designer is to avoid harm to the actor who plays the *Christus* character as he hangs on the cross, the raw fact is that he has to stay up there for thirty-five minutes.

Over the years the play has garnered severe criticism for its anti-Semitic attacks. The script for 2000 excised the offending language. No longer need one be a baptized Christian to participate. It stands for Christians as a great statement of faith. For non-Christians it is a splendid dramatization of a heroic story.

Professionally, I found much to admire. The orchestral and choral music, all live, was splendid. Sets, costumes, lighting, and staging were spectacular. I have heard that the play had been rather amateurish in the past. If so, no longer. It would withstand professional scrutiny from any angle.

For me, the experience held me to account for my own faith, my own dedication. Is there anything to which I would totally dedicate myself?

CHAPTER 34

SANDY RIVERS

Sandy Rivers was a good acquaintance, though not a close friend. I enjoyed meeting Sandy at social events. We usually had things to talk about: basketball, opera, movies. Sandy is a nickname for Sandor. The name also applied to his hair, but he had detested the nickname as a child. "Kids teased me that my real name was Sandra" Another point of contact. When I was a boy, I heard, "Carroll is a girl," too many times. But then Sandy had learned about Sandy Koufax, and decided that his name was okay.

I managed my own brand of teasing. "How are the rivers today? Rocky? Smooth? Swift? Sandy?"

He might have a quick retort. "Well, *Carolus*, I wouldn't go *Roman* in swift waters."

We had never stayed on a serious subject more than a couple of minutes without moving into wisecracking. He usually won.

That's why the card surprised me so.

It was a Snoopy card, with a picture of Snoopy in his "vulture" pose on the front of it. The cover caption read, "Here's the vulture trying to scare all your troubles away." The inside caption: "I hope it works soon. I'm starting to feel ridiculous." I laughed at the card, then read Sandy's note.

"Carolus, my 'Roman' friend, I just heard about your radiation. I understand the PSA did a big jump after radiation. We have been dealing with prostate cancer with my father-in-law. Please know that you and Clarice are in our prayers. Also, pray for Lori and me. It works both ways, you know!"

I called Sandy and suggested we get together for lunch. We met at Applebee's. He talked about his concerns for Lori's dad. He listened attentively to my story, interjecting probing questions. We met for lunch several times over the next few months. I began to appreciate Sandy as a man of deep faith and spiritual insight. I even dared to share some of my dreams with him. We promised to keep praying for each other. We also kept up our running rule of mandatory wise-cracking.

"Sir Sandor, how the hell are you?"

"About the fifth level down, Carolus."

Lori and Clarice seemed to think our friendship was good for all of us. We each had another guy we could "dump" on, taking some emotional pressure off of our wives. As the months passed, we became involved in other things and let our lunch visits slide. Once in a while, I would call, or we would meet at a social function.

It was a Saturday night. Clarice and I were both home. The phone rang. It was Sandy. "Put Clarice on the line too. I want you both to hear this at the same time." I sensed this was not a time for wisecracks. "I want you to be among the first to know that I have bilateral testicular cancer."

I sat with Lori during Sandy's surgery. He had radiation. He had chemo. We got reports that he was doing well. But I never heard directly from Sandy or Lori. I sent cards. I called every few weeks. I always got their voice mail. He never returned my calls. I had let him and Lori read parts of my chronicle, so I sent new chapters to him. I took a letter, with two recent chapters of *Journey toward Wholeness,* to his office. He was not in. I instructed his secretary that the package was an important correspondence.

The letter gave him an update on my situation and asked him to fill me in on his.

Silence.

I was puzzled. I was hurt. A friend had walked out of my life without saying good-bye. A mutual friend told Clarice that Sandy was having a rough time dealing with his illness. I thought, *That's what friends are for!*

I made a couple more calls. Voice mail. No reply. I gave up.

Many months later Clarice received an e-mail describing kinds of friends. "Some friends are friends for a reason. Some are friends for a season. Some are friends forever." She said: "Maybe this will help you understand Sandy. He was a friend for a season, and a reason. You gave each other support when it was most needed. Then the friendship had served its purpose, and you each moved on."

Maybe so. But I still missed seeing the only person who called me Carolus.

CHAPTER 35

THE NEXT BRICK FALLS

I feel like I've lost two whole weeks out of my life." Saturday, March 17, 2001. St. Patrick's Day. Late afternoon. Clarice and I had just returned from a trip to Southern Indiana, a day spent judging a choir contest.

"Honey, it's been three weeks."

"What? It can't be!" I checked the calendar. Sure enough. From February 24 to March 17 is three weeks.

Three Saturdays before, Clarice and I both had served as judges for the Indiana State School Music Association solo vocal contest. State contest is a big event running over two weekends: instrumental one week, vocal and piano the next. We were among forty judges adjudicating nearly two thousand vocal events. Clarice spent the day listening to fifty female vocal soloists. I heard fifty male singers. Performers coming to state contest have already earned a first division (top rating) in group 1, the most demanding, at their district level. They pour into Indianapolis by car, van, and bus from all around the state. Each soloist has six minutes to sing one song, for the reward of a professional evaluation and the chance to earn a medal. We both enjoy the chance to hear well-prepared, earnest young performers at their best. We both try to give each performer a complete, honest, encouraging, and instructive evaluation. The work is intense and fun.

We decided to get an early dinner before heading home, so we tried out a new "gourmet burger" place that promised perfect charbroiled hamburgers prepared with all-fresh fixings. When we got home, I fed the animals and took Prince, the yellow Labrador, for a walk. As I walked, I developed the worst heartburn I had ever experienced. Along with it came deep-down-in-the-belly hiccups and belching that seemed to come from my toes. Belching and hiccuping at the same time puts something of a strain on the lower abs. I kept walking. Several laps with the Lab around the condos, trying deep breathing, holding my breath, and stretching. After maybe twenty minutes, the convulsions had calmed enough that I could enter the house without shaking the chandelier.

Clarice claims that my hiccups are strong enough to rattle the windows. They have lasted, usually at times of great stress, for as long as three days. She discovered my Vesuvian capacities when I visited her parents for the first time. I have learned all the folk cures, including one she tried to teach me years ago at her parents' house when she instructed me to "breathe into a paper bag." I dutifully found a paper bag and tried to do as told. She and her mother broke into fits of laughter when I came into the kitchen with the bag over my head.

The easiest, and most effective, solution for me: hold a mouthful of water in your mouth, close your nostrils and ears with your fingers, and swallow the water slowly. On this February evening, I tried the cure as soon as I got back into the house. It helped. For maybe a half hour.

Then the whole thing started again.

We had decided to watch the video of *My Fair Lady* that evening. As we watched the movie, the spasms calmed down, leaving my lower abs feeling sore and overworked. Then a dull pain emerged near the groin. "Oh, no! Not a pulled groin muscle!"

The pain intensified. By the time I got ready for bed, I could find no comfortable position. I took a couple of Tylenol and tried to relax. The bed was no good. The recliner did not work. The sofa offered no comfort. The floor worked only if I curled up in a fetal position. I tried walking around. The pain got worse. About midnight I felt a wave of nausea.

Usually I will do anything to keep from throwing up, but this time I begged for it to come. Six times during the night, I made the dash. Clarice slept through the whole thing. At 1:00, 3:00, and 5:00, I almost woke her up, but thought, "No. I can make it until morning." By now I figured that maybe I had a twisted or impacted bowel. *Don't horses with twisted bowels have to be shot?* I became dizzy and broke into a cold sweat when I tried to walk.

At six in the morning, I knew I could no longer wait. "Honey, I think I need you to take me to the emergency room. But don't rush. Go ahead and get ready for church." I figured she could drop me off at the ER, go to church, and come back later. While she got dressed, I finally slept. When she was ready to leave at 7:00, I was out of pain.

I said: "The emergency seems to be over. Go ahead to church. If I have to go, I'll drive myself to the emergency room."

"Oh, no, you won't! You'll call 911 and let an ambulance take you. You're not going to drive if you are in the condition you were in last night."

I know when the Boss is in charge. "Yes, Ma'am." Then off to sleep I drifted.

I got up around eleven, feeling refreshed. Took a shower. Read the paper. When Clarice got home, I started to fix lunch. As I stood at the kitchen counter mixing the soup, a knife stabbed me in the groin. "I think we'd better make that hospital trip."

Some of my thoughts from the long night came back to me. "I remember Dr. Schick instructing as to how I would know if the cancer got into the bones. His answer was, 'Pain. Intense, unrelenting pain.'

"I also wonder if the abdominal spasms have maybe shaken up an undiscovered tumor that is blocking the bowel."

Her instinctive protective shield flew up. "Don't even think about it!" she shot out. I realized she was more frightened than I was, although she claimed she was trying to keep me from thinking negative thoughts. I decided to keep my darker thoughts to myself for a while. She helped me into the car, and I laid the seat back. We had just gotten a new Honda Accord. I had been bragging about its quiet, smooth ride. But on our eight-mile trip to the hospital, I felt every chuckhole, every groove, every pebble in the road.

The triage nurse interviewed me within two minutes of our arrival. Soon the ER doctor came in. He ordered an EKG and several other tests. He said, "I'm going to have to check your privates."

Come on, man! Didn't they teach you proper anatomical terms in med school?

When I tried to shift my weight on the gurney, the pain made me cry out. I started hyperventilating and sobbing. Clarice calmly informed the doctor, "Panic attack." *Not this time. This is Pain with a capital P and that rhymes with D and that stands for "Don't touch me."*

But he did it anyway. He touched my left testicle. It felt like a 220-volt shock. He promised some morphine and Valium. Two doses of morphine didn't touch the pain.

He found nothing abnormal in the testicles. The doctor explained that often the location of touch sensitivity is not the origin of the problem. A problem occurring along one portion of a nerve can relay the sensation of pain elsewhere. He called it a "referred pain."

Finally, a dose of Vicodin brought some relief, sixteen hours after the pain started. The ER doctor could find nothing, so he ordered more Vicodin and urged me to see Dr. Shiller or Dr. Logan the next day. Loaded down with Vicodin, I slept well that night.

CHAPTER 36

INVASION

On Monday I cancelled all my appointments and took myself to Dr. Logan. I said: "I don't know whether you are the person I need to see or not. The pain seems to center around the lower abdomen and testicles. Dr. Shiller is the 'nut' doctor. But you're the one I could get in to see." He examined the charts from the ER, ran more tests, and found nothing. A consultation with Dr. Logan is like sitting in a med school class. He rapidly counted off maybe a dozen things that could be suspects, and just as rapidly ruled them out. He ordered a CT scan for the next morning.

His nurse gave me a barium "milkshake" to drink at bedtime. At 7:00 Tuesday morning, Clarice took me to the lab and waited for me. By 8:00 we were done. But I could tell that I would be no good for any activity. "Honey, can you take my rehearsal this morning?" My women's chorus meets every Tuesday morning. Clarice, having been their director for several seasons, knows them well. Taking my rehearsal meant losing work for her. She arranged for a half day off of work, left me to crawl back into bed, and set out to whip "my ladies" into shape.

By Wednesday the Vicodin was letting me feel almost normal. Dr. Logan called with the report on the CT scan. Lymph nodes around the right ureter (leading from the kidney to the bladder) had become enlarged. They were squeezing in on the ureter. So the source of the pain was a blocked kidney. Dr. Logan made an appointment for me to see Dr.

Shiller to have a stent inserted into the ureter. The stent would keep it open so urine could flow freely. The stent was a stopgap to keep me going until we could shrink the lymph nodes. Dr. Logan did not deem it necessary to biopsy the lymph nodes. "To do a biopsy in that area would be a very invasive procedure. Besides, it is not necessary. We have the evidence: (a) prostate cancer, (b) elevated PSA, (c) enlarged lymph nodes. Prostate cancer goes most directly to the lymph nodes. The treatment will be the same with or without a biopsy."

Our church handbell choir was to play for a community Ash Wednesday service at Witherspoon Presbyterian Church. Paula White, bell ringer and soprano extraordinaire, also has a truck. She and I transported the bell equipment. I kept feeling little tugs in the lower abdomen as I lifted bell cases and tables, but thanks to being drugged, I avoided the intense pain of the past Sunday. For the service our bells played "Just a Closer Walk with Thee":

> I am weak, but thou art strong.
> Keep me, Jesus, from all wrong.
> I'll be satisfied as long
> As I walk, precious Lord, close to Thee.
> Just a closer walk with Thee,
> Grant it, Jesus, is my plea,
> Daily walking close to Thee
> Let it be, dear Lord, let it be.[59]

The words and music went straight to my soul.

On Thursday I had an early-morning consultation with Dr. Shiller. He showed me a stent, a plastic tube about eighteen inches long. He would run it up through my penis, through the urethra, past the bladder, through the ureter, and into the kidney. It was the same procedure as a plumbing "snake." One end would curl up in the kidney, the other in the bladder. I said, "Any messing around with that part of my anatomy, I don't want to know about."

Wednesday's exertion, along with that news, took its toll. I cancelled Thursday lessons, but geared myself up to attend our Stephen Ministry meeting that evening. Among people whom I know and trust, I can get a little zany, but I think the journal entry I shared with them that night sent my most trusted friends reeling.

The Ole Boy 03-01-2001
He hunches forward in his Barcalounger,
elbows on his knees.
Hanging loosely in his left hand
a half-eaten The Works pizza,
in the other, a warm bottle of Bud Heavy.
He stares at the floor.
He shakes his head.
"Well, boys, it's time you knew:
It's the Ole Big C."
Looks as close to reverential dismay
as bleary-eyed boozers can conjure up
encircle him.
They huddle closer—
don't look him in the eye—
that's for enemies, not friends.
Finally one speaks,
"So, Duke, whatcha gonna do?"
Duke had thought about it.
"Te' ye' whut, Earl.
I've seen many ole rattlesnake
curled up in the sage brush,
jes' waitin' t' strike.
But me, I wuz alles faster.
My trusty Colt .45
'd git 'im b'tween th' eyes
afore 'e could strike."
The big screen TV across the room
was showing gaudy, expensive cars
tumbling over each other.
Earl nodded his head like he knew
what Duke was talking about,

but he was really watching
how that Chevy flipped over,
come upright,
and kept going.
"Y'know, Duke,
yer gonna be like that Chevy.
Yer gonna land on yer wheels an' keep goin'."
A commercial came on.
The one with the frogs.
Any reptile or amphibian was close enough
to being a rattlesnake to enrage Duke.
He looked at his hands—
Pizza in the left.
Beer in the right.
He hauled back and hurled.
He forgot he was left-handed—
A splatter of tomatoes,
mushrooms,
pepperoni,
sausage,
and anchovies
caught that frog right in the face.

Amee listened to the whole thing with saucer-eyes. She laughed the laugh of someone who doesn't believe what she has just heard. "Where—where did that come from? I've read a lot of your writing, but never anything like this!"

I really did not know. "Well, it's sort of a guy thinking what a gal might think a guy is thinking." I thought about it some more on the way home. My rational brain had no real explanation. I began feeling uncertain. I read it to Clarice, who laughed, relieving some of my uncertainty.

Then she asked, "What *were* you trying to say?"

It hit me. "This was my way of tackling my fear and anger: standing up to the thing that scares me most and throwing a pizza in its face."

"I'm glad you found a way to bring out your fear and anger."

✳

On Friday afternoon I reported to the Surgery Center for the stent placement. Clarice went with me as the nurse led me to a cozy little prep room set up like a small den. I lounged in a recliner while the nurse took my vitals and started an IV. The anesthesiologist came in and explained the medications he would give me. "We'll put an adhesive strip on your forehead. It will read how deeply asleep you are. That way we know exactly how much anesthesia to give you." The nurse walked me back to the surgery room. The anesthesiologist activated the sedation drip, then started asking me questions. "Where do you work? Where did you go to school?" By the third question, I was gone.

Two hours later I was on the way home, without that awful pressure I had felt on the ureter for several days. I knew the stent was a stopgap; we had to reduce the swelling. I also knew it was temporary. Dr. Shiller said he would need to replace it about every three months. I determined to get the swollen lymph nodes under control before he would have to put in another stent.

Saturday morning Clarice drove me to St. Luke's United Methodist Church for a regional Stephen Ministry workshop. Amee and one other person from Saint Andrew also attended. I managed the morning without any mishaps, but asked Amee to take me home after lunch. I slept most of the afternoon.

I knew it would take several days to get over the anesthesia. I talked to Joi on the phone. She reminded me that people with more body fat take longer to shake off anesthesia than do people with little body fat. Thanks, dear daughter. I managed the next couple of days by keeping a light schedule. At the next Tuesday rehearsal with my women's chorus, the ladies formed a prayer circle to pray for me.

That afternoon Joi and Emily arrived for the last "prenatal" visit before Joi's second baby was due. She immediately took off for a night out with her friends, leaving Clarice and me to baby-sit with the granddaughter.

On Wednesday, March 7, I did my monthly radio appearance as storyteller in residence at WICR-FM. Paul, the host, told the radio audience that I was to have a bone scan and further tests. He told me on the air: "I'm about to choke up. You bring so much to us. You are such a good friend." I was startled to hear such personal words going out over the air.

That afternoon I had a message on my phone from Miriam, the organist at Downey Avenue Christian Church, where I had been choir director for eight years. "I heard you on the radio this morning, and heard Paul say that you had some continuing health concerns. Please call me and fill me in so I can tell the choir. You are in all our prayers."

As much as I loved having Joi and Emily here, I had to excuse myself to nap several times during their visit. Finally, by Saturday I worked up enough energy to play with Emily—doing "skinny-cats," dancing, getting down on the floor, and playing tag—things granddads are made for.

Anxiety over the impending bone scan report impaired my function for most of the next week. At Broad Ripple High School, students were taking standardized tests. Because the normal class schedule was upset, I had carefully worked out a teaching schedule that would get me some time with each private student. Seeing my physical and emotional state, Alice, my supervisor, said, "Why don't you just take the week off?" So I did. I tried to keep my lessons at my private studio, but had to cancel some of them, also.

Thursday, the Ides of March. Clarice met me at Dr. Logan's office for a report on the bone scan and a treatment-planning session. The bone scan report indicated suspicious areas in the sacrum (the large triangular bone in the lower spine) and in the sacroiliac (the connection between the two sides of the sacrum). The report said that this finding was "worrisome for metastasis." Now we had abnormal activity in lymph nodes and bones. Time for action.

Dr. Logan reminded me that my subjective reaction to the standard hormonal treatment had been the worst he had ever seen.

"Thanks. I like to break records, but not that kind."

He would not recommend returning to the Lupron and Casodex. Prednisone could reduce swelling, but probably would not affect the PSA. It was too early for chemotherapy. Bilateral orchiectomy (castration) would be an option, but he did not recommend it. Other treatments one can change or reverse. Once the testicles are removed, they can't be put back. With castration, I would also experience the same testosterone-deprivation symptoms that I had with the Lupron.

I said: "Earlier you mentioned Premarin. Is that still an option?"

"Yes. We don't have clinical studies on it, but I have used it, and it is effective. I don't know what a proper dose would be."

"I am willing to start with a low dose and keep increasing it until it has some effect. Clarice takes it with no ill effects." Premarin is an estrogen-replacement drug that postmenopausal women take to prevent osteoporosis. "You will be taking more than she takes." He left the room to consult his manual. He returned. "I'll be glad to prescribe Premarin. It will be three, 1.25 mg tablets a day to start with." That is six times the dosage Clarice takes for hormone replacement.

"The pharmacist may look at you funny. You may have to explain that you are not doing a sex change! But you should never have any trouble with osteoporosis. This stuff will make your bones like iron!"[60]

I asked again about side effects.

"You may carry some risk of heart disease or phlebitis, but I would rather run the slight risk of heart trouble than the sure promise of advancing prostate cancer. You may also experience enlargement of the breasts.

"I'm going to set you up with Dr. Schick, the radiologist, to arrange for spot radiation to prevent breast enlargement and to bring down the swelling of the lymph nodes."

Now we had a course of action. Much of my upset stomach and anxiety eased up. That evening I called Joel, Joi, and Jon to give them the report. Jeremy was temporarily in Louisville, and we did not have a phone number for him. Joel said: "You have had so much to overcome. I don't know how you handle it. I know I couldn't deal with something like that." I feel strange hearing things like that from my brother. I have, from boyhood, looked up to him as the strong member of our family.

Jon was in New Orleans on business. I called his cell phone. He answered immediately. "Oh, hi, Dad!"

"Jon, are you in a night club? I hear a trombone playing 'Sweet Georgia Brown' in the background."

"No. I'm on Bourbon Street!" The wonders of the wireless age.

※

Saturday came, St. Paddy's Day, and the realization that three weeks had passed since my attack. I had been unconscious much of the time, stumbling through the mechanics of duties part of the time. Some events I recalled later as if I had dreamed them.

Sunday I had to go to church, even though I still felt groggy. The handbells were playing, and I was covering two bass bell positions. As I walked toward the sanctuary, I saw Amee and her husband, Sven. She gave me a big hug. "Clarice told us your news. Premarin and radiation? Are they going to zap your boobs?"

"Yep. I don't want to have to be fitted for a bra."

This conversation was with a woman who had undergone a double mastectomy.

Monday called me back to a more-than-full schedule at the high school. Nearly half of my students had missed three weeks of lessons—lessons that I was obligated to make up. Time had arrived for a full health disclosure. I had never kept my cancer a secret, or avoided questions. Yet I had made no public announcements. As I met each student, I explained why I had been absent. For the younger ones, I gave no details. For the juniors and seniors whom I knew well, I filled in details as they asked. A young woman who has health problems of her own gave me a card. "Dr. Stegall, I still can't believe that you never told us about your cancer, and here I am worrying about my silly problems. I was terribly glad to see you in good health after I heard. I hope you get better, because you have been a wonderful teacher and I wouldn't like you to stop."

Now that the disease was "outed," I figured that if I caught a cold, which I did, impressionable teenagers would suspect the worst. I felt more pressure than before to "put on a good face."

My Wednesday visit with Dr. Schick would be, I thought, rather straightforward. Instead, he presented more complications. I had hoped that the radiation treatment could be short. "No. We have to do a full, thirty-treatment series. Anytime we shoot into the abdomen, we have to use small doses to protect the other organs." That's six weeks of treatments at five days a week. I remembered how the full treatment had debilitated me five years earlier.

"Most men who die of prostate cancer die because the cancer replaces bone marrow, depleting the body of red blood cells. If we radiate the bones, we will also destroy bone marrow. We do have erythropoietin, which stimulates bone marrow growth. However, it may simply provide more food for the cancer to feed on.

Dr. Schick continued, "Eventually we will get bone metastasis. Can we get by without radiation for now? Can we just change the stent as necessary until something new develops?"

My question about whether Premarin itself might reduce the lymph swelling got a dubious "maybe."

Acknowledging that mine "is a complex case," he urged me to bring Clarice with me the following week, when we would decide for sure what to do about the lymph and bone radiation. He would radiate the breasts in preparation for taking Premarin in any case. He told me that a new drug, Zofran, would ease any nausea I might experience.

He assured me that the same treatment would target the bones and the lymph nodes. "We don't have to give double doses. One shot serves both purposes, because they are in line with each other."

A week later Clarice went with me for my pre-radiation consultation. I told her that Dr. Schick would set up the procedure and the techs would carry out the therapy. I remembered that they were tuned in to the patient's discomfort, and made the therapy as low-stress as possible. "A couple of the girls loved flirting."

"Well, they better watch out how they flirt!"

Jennifer, the head radiation technologist, came into the examining room. She remembered me from my treatments five years earlier. She winked, gave a little grin, touched her hand to my knee, and said, "We're going to take good care of you."

I turned to Clarice. "She's one of the flirters."

Jennifer pretended to be indignant. "I don't flirt! We're just old friends!"

She went over the routine for the CT scan I would have the next day. She wrote on the instructions that I would go to the "Proffesional Building."

"Neat spelling," I chided. "Two *f*s and one *s*."

"Oh, cut that out! I know how it's spelled. Would you believe that I was the best speller in my class in school?"

"Sure. And I want to make sure I have your name right: J-e-n-i-f-f-e-r, with one *n* and two *f*s. Got it."

"You're never going to let me live down that goof, are you?"

I think Clarice could understand why I had not minded too much the daily pilgrimage to the Cancer Center when I had to go.

CHAPTER 37

THE OWL

I had to whack holes in my teaching schedule to arrange for the CT scan on Thursday. Then came another trip on Friday for simulation: X rays, lining up angles, painting gun sights on my abdomen. By late Thursday afternoon, I felt apprehension and anxiety creeping in around my brain. When I took Prince out for his evening walk, I started stumbling and hyperventilating.

Then I heard the owl. I had not heard him since fall. I had never seen him. Sometimes, even inside our condo with the windows closed, we can hear him and his mate call to each other. Anytime we hear them, we stop whatever we are doing, ease our way out onto the patio, listen, and watch.

Once when Jeremy was walking Prince at night, he heard them calling back and forth. Then he looked up and saw them both swoop silently down the path, just a few feet over his head—a diversion practice to keep any intruders away from the nest. "Their wingspan was at least four feet," he reported. The silence of their flight, coupled with their sudden appearance, daring to come within a few feet of my son's head, enhanced the mystery as well as the reality of those invisible night hunters.

Another time, when Joi and her family were visiting, I took Prince and two-year-old Emily for a walk in the woods. Emily was confident. "Prince show us owl." We watched and waited, silent. Emily became solemn. "I don't see the owl."

I hope Emily does get to hear it. I hope she gets to see it, though I fear that intruding "development" has chased the owls away. But she has heard it and seen it through the ears and eyes of her mind. It was the greatest owl she never saw.

Now, on a March walk with Prince, I heard the owl again. I stopped to listen. I had always heard the voice coming from the same place in the little wooded area behind our condo. I stopped to listen. There was that call again. Whoo - Whoo - wh-wh-wh- Whoo - *Whoo* - Whoo. Two notes on E-flat, rising through E-natural and F to G-flat for the last three notes. I answered and listened. He called back.

Then I saw him.

He was perched on the end of a nearly vertical dead branch. In the early evening mist, he looked like an extension of the branch. The first sliver of the new moon arched just over his head.

I let Prince roam in the woods while I watched. I called again. His answer this time put a trill on the last three notes. I answered, imitating his trill. He turned his head my way. The peaked tufts told me: a great horned owl. I swear he saw me in the gathering dusk. We called back and forth several times. When he trilled his last three notes, so did I. When he sang them straight, so did I.

He spread his wings and swooped away, hardly moving his wings. Totally silent in flight. Wingspan of maybe four feet. He perched on a nearby tree. He called again. So did I. I called Prince. I flew on my own silent wings back to the house. "Honey! I saw the owl! He sang back to me!"

"I know. I heard you out there, calling to him."

Now I was ready for whatever the meds wanted to throw at me. Or so I thought.

Friday morning at 8:00, I presented myself to the Cancer Center for simulation. Jennifer was waiting at the door for me with her "Welcome, friend" grin. Dr. Schick rushed in with a report from the CT scan taken the day before. He was in a hurry. "I have to be at the eastside clinic for a 9:00 seed implantation." He then hit me with the bad news, based on the latest pictures. Radiation may be harmful and may not accomplish the needed therapy. The CT scan showed enlarged lymph nodes overlapping the prostate bed. Shooting through the same tissues he had irradiated five years earlier could cause irreparable damage. "I recall that you had a terrible time with the radiation then. That's nothing to what it could be if we damage your colon."

That wasn't all. "Even if we can shrink the lymph nodes that are squeezing on the ureter, they could shrivel up and actually squeeze tighter. We may also have scar tissue forming in the ureter itself.

"You know I wasn't wild about doing the treatment in the first place. With this new information, I strongly recommend against it. I swear to you, if you were my brother, I would say, 'don't do it.'"

I asked him to go over it again to make sure I understood it clearly.

"Carroll, look. I have two minutes. Let us set up the breast radiation and talk about the extended treatment when I get back from vacation in two weeks."

I wasn't accustomed to any of my doctors cutting me off. I knew he did not want to be abrupt, but I still felt like I had been slapped.

I was trembling inside when Jennifer and her assistant returned to take measurements for the breast radiation. I faced Jennifer. "Does it seem strange that I am disappointed that Dr. Schick does not want to radiate?"

"No. Not at all."

For the first time, I felt like the disease was controlling me. If I rushed, I could have made it to school in time to catch my first voice student. Instead I went to the bank, gassed up my car, bought a Krispy Kreme doughnut, and headed for Clarice's office. I wanted to tell her face-to-face. She acted calm. We held each other in a long embrace.

One of her coworkers walked past her office. She stuck her head in the door. "Now, now! No fraternizing on company time! I swear you two act like newlyweds!"

At school, it was the last day before spring break. No one wanted to be in class. Time to kick back and visit. The rest of the day was incredibly full, with rich personal sharing with colleagues and students.

I was nearly through reading a novel that Clarice had passed on to me. Not great literature, but a gripping story of alienation and reconciliation. That afternoon she and I both had appointments with Cheri, the delightful French lady who has been our hairdresser for several years. My appointment was first. Cheri, petite and suave, even though she is of my generation, looks just right in leather hip-hugger slacks and platform shoes.

Cheri and I talked about her husband, who has leukemia. He is a robust man who does not trust doctors and won't talk about his illness. His pain and depression have forced Cheri to take antidepressants to cope with him. They both sense that they don't have a lot of time left together. He shows his fear through impatience and anger.

While Cheri worked on Clarice's hair, I finished the novel and offered it to Cheri to read. One theme of the story is that important things left unsaid can destroy you. Some of the characters learn. Others don't.

Clarice and I were planning to see a movie that evening. Cheri said, "You must see *Chocolat!* You will experience bigotry and prejudice, and how one person overcomes it. The photography is beautiful. It was filmed in a village like the one where I grew up. And—you will come out craving chocolate!"

So *Chocolat* it was. Cheri was right on all counts.

After the film we returned home, glowing from the simple story of alienation and reconciliation we had just seen on the screen. I brought in the mail. In the stack of flyers and credit card offers was a letter addressed to R.C.S. A real letter from our youngest child, currently living in Knoxville. I knew it would not be a casual greeting. I sat down at the kitchen table and started reading.

His typical square-block printing, in tiny letters, perfectly straight on ruled yellow legal paper, filled five pages. By the second page, I was sobbing. Clarice eased over and gripped my shoulder while I read. My body shook with sobs. My eyes flooded. I wailed.

"What is it?" Her voice was gentle, soothing.

"It's so wonderful—I can't believe what I'm reading." Our rebellious son was telling me how much he loved me.

When I got through, she asked, "May I read it?"

I guided her to the sofa. "Read it to me. Aloud."

I laid my head on her shoulder as she read, in part, "The news on your health frightens me and worries me. The first: as a boy, you were always a giant to me, the strongest man alive; now I am frightened that another giant will take you away from me. The second: I am worried that I have squandered our time together by not getting to know you better. You, the only man to have loved me unconditionally since the day sun first shone on my face."

I wanted to talk to my son, but I thought I would break down if I called him right then. Immediately the phone rang. It was my son. Clarice chatted with him long enough for me to compose myself. I gave him the medical update, then I said: "Three very important things happened today. I finished a book about reconciliation. We saw a movie about reconciliation. Then I got a letter about reconciliation."

I could hear him crying as I told him how moved I was and how I cherished his letter. We talked for about fifteen minutes and said good-bye.

As soon as we hung up, I remembered something important.

I immediately called him back and told him about the owl.

CHAPTER 38

PLAYING "WHAT IF?"

Tonight we are examining new procedures in remote brachytherapy. Our presenter, Dr. Harvey Schick, is president of the American College of Radiation Oncologists. Before Dr. Schick begins, he would like to hear each of you tell a little about your case." Dick, the convener for the support group meeting, then opened the floor for members of the group to speak.

"I was diagnosed in 1998, had a PSA of 14, underwent a radical prostatectomy and follow-up radiation. My PSA reads .0001 at present."

"I had a radioactive seed implantation in 1996, am on Lupron and Casodex. I feel great. My PSA is 3.1, holding steady."

"I had a radical in 1999. Dr. Schick followed up with radiation. My PSA is zero."

"After a radical in 1997, I had radiation with Dr. Schick. In 1998 my PSA went to 97, so I started Lupron and Casodex. I'm now at 2.1 and feel good."

Around the room came the reports. Radical prostatectomy, radioactive seed implantation, radiation, chemotherapy, hormone treatment. All under control.

My turn came. "I had a radical in 1995. Dr. Schick directed follow-up radiation. Dr. Schick must not have done a very good job, because my PSA jumped to 95 during radiation." Chuckles around the room. "I took Lupron and Casodex off and on for three years. I did not tolerate them well. The PSA remained in check throughout most of 2000 without hormone treatment, then jumped to 528 in October. In March 2001 we discovered enlarged lymph nodes and spots on my tailbone. Dr. Schick didn't think it safe to radiate, so I'm now on megadoses of Premarin. Anybody here take Premarin?"

None of the men raised their hands.

All the women did.

The audience laughed.

Dr. Schick is on the leading edge of new radiation therapies. His spiffy PowerPoint display showed the difference between what an MRI or a CT scan could show a year before, and what it revealed now. The difference was that of walking into a room at night with only moonlight filtering through the curtain, then turning on the lights.

The new treatment permits him to aim short, powerful doses of radiation in precise quantities to specific locations, all monitored by real-time ultrasound images. He can even control the release pattern of a specific dose to fit the shape and size of the tissue he is targeting. At the time of his July 2001 presentation, he had treated just four men with the new procedure. Early results indicated minimal damage to healthy tissue, no loss of potency, and no incontinence.

Dr. Schick spoke to me after the presentation. He acted, as always, very solicitous. "You know, Carroll, if we had had the precision measurements five years ago that we have now, I probably could have gotten it all."

I answered: "But we're not playing 'what if.' You did the best job anybody could do in 1996. It just underscores how far medicine has come in such a short time."

I called Jon and told him about the new treatment. I knew that Jon was fascinated by new technologies. I said, "I'm still hoping to get *Journey toward Wholeness* published. I realize how outdated the treatments are that I had five years ago. Perhaps I should cut way back on the medical descriptions, since they are no longer applicable."

"I don't know, Dad. I think that if people read about what you have survived, and realize how medicine has advanced, it will give them hope."

Jon's reply gave me a new way of seeing. Just like the time when he was in high school and we got into a shouting match over a *Macbeth* assignment, and I came out of it with a whole new focus on the play that I thought I knew so well.

My first treatment was the most advanced available in 1995. Dr. Shiller had the technique for the least invasive surgery possible. Dr. Schick had the latest in external beam radiation, with targeting and dosage control much advanced over what was available anywhere else in the state at the time. Mine was the first prescription of Casodex that my pharmacy filled.

The new treatment I started in April 2001 is actually a throwback to an earlier treatment that was being abandoned at about the time that I started my hormone therapy.

There are two basic approaches to hormone therapy for prostate cancer. The first is to introduce a competitor. Large doses of estrogen will compete with testosterone for the hormone receptors in each cell, rendering testosterone ineffective as a food source for the prostate cancer.

The second approach is to shut off testosterone production. That is what we had tried the first time around, with Lupron and Casodex. It made me feel awful. Yet when it maintained effectiveness for four years (counting the one year with no treatment), I had already beaten the odds. When I began Lupron and Casodex, Dr. Shiller told me we could expect it to work for eighteen to twenty-four months.

When Dr. Logan introduced me to Premarin in March 2001, he was returning to the first, earlier approach, using a drug that was developed for other purposes. Premarin, a form of estrogen, is designed for hormone replacement in postmenopausal women. For a number of years, the preferred hormone therapy for prostate cancer was DES, the estrogen product that Eli Lilly took off the market in 1997.[61]

My Premarin dosage was six times what Clarice takes.

In the first seventeen weeks after starting Premarin, my PSA dropped 82 percent, a startling three points per day. At the same time, I had greatly increased energy. Sometimes I would get hyper, then wear out. I might get too agitated to sleep, then have trouble waking up. Those developments led to my determination to increase my vigilance regarding regular sleeping hours, exercise, and a moderate low-fat diet. Depression and anxiety became milder and less frequent, yet with some dramatic lapses.

CHAPTER 39

AT JUST THE RIGHT MOMENT

For several weeks after talking with Dr. Schick, I maintained good energy and refreshing sleep, getting many needed projects done around the house that I would not have time to do when school started.

On a Wednesday afternoon in August, after returning home from a meeting, I ate lunch and worked on the daily crossword puzzle, then stretched out in the Barcalounger our son had brought over from his workplace. Toonces, our Siamese-tabby, jumped up onto my chest and set in to heavy purring. I was about to doze off when a thought jolted me awake. "I need to organize my tools in the garage." Our son had recently cleared his furniture from the garage. I had intended to get my things in order as soon as he had made room. I jumped up, opened the garage door, and set up my worktable. Part of my garage organization project was to clean, oil, and inventory all our antique and heirloom tools, then to store all the small ones in my large metal toolbox. With that project complete, our children would know which handsaw belonged to Daddy, which to Clarice's dad, and which to Uncle Charley.

Just as I began laying out the tools, a new Grand Am slowed down and stopped at the end of my driveway. The window rolled down. I heard a voice. "Carroll?" I looked up and saw a man getting out of the car. It was John Schild, one of my Maennerchor friends. I met him halfway down the short driveway, where we gave each other bear hugs.

"What brings you out here?"

"A man who works for me lives in this complex. I was checking in on him."

"Did you know we were living here?"

"I knew you were out here somewhere, but didn't know which building."

Had I not been in my open garage, he would have passed me by. I invited him in. I had some important matters of family, career, and faith that I needed to talk about. I was able to share with him some events in our lives that neither Clarice nor I was free to discuss with our other friends. John had come by at just the right moment. I do not believe that the impulse to go out and open the garage was mere happenstance. Especially since I love my naps so much.

On Saturday I finished the garage and some other home projects, cleaned up, and headed to a hair appointment. I always look forward to having Cheri work on my hair and to our conversations. This day she told me about her grandparents who helped raise her in their little home village in the French Alps. "My grandfather was seven feet tall. My grandmother was barely five feet. When I was a little girl and got hurt, my grandmother would cradle me in her lap and comfort me. When I came to America and ran into difficult times, I cried for my grandmother, but she was already gone."

She continued: "One night I went down to my basement and started painting. I painted a background of the Alps, shrouded in mist. Then I put in our village with snow on the ground. In the foreground I painted an old woman holding a little girl. The little girl was me, though I was a grown woman when I painted it. That picture got me through those hard times."

"You still have that painting, I bet."

Her scissors kept up their rhythmic clicking. "I would never part with it for a million dollars. It is my connection with my ancestors." She paused, stopped clipping, and walked around to face me. "I don't know why I tell you these things. I don't talk about my personal life. We French guard our privacy. It takes us a long time to develop close friends."

Then she gave me a vigorous neck and shoulder massage, a privilege she reserves for her male customers. I always come away from my hair appointments feeling like my life is worthwhile.

Still glowing from that visit, I headed across town for my appointed meeting with my Stephen Ministry care receiver. His wife was leaving to run errands when I arrived. She served me a glass of ice water as I sat down in one of their matching recliners. My care receiver took the other chair. On this day he had some life-changing events to consider. He was nearly eighty, with multiple health problems. He and his devoted wife had raised all their children in this house. They had seen the children all marry, establish careers, and have children of their own. A lifetime of memories infused that house. Now the rest of the family were urging Mom and Dad to move into a retirement community, a heart-wrenching prospect for him. I listened and asked questions for two hours as he spun stories of life in their house, telling me what year he planted each tree.

"Gardening is your great love, isn't it?"

"And fishing. But fishing is a long-past memory now. I haven't taken the boat out in six years. I have it being fixed up to sell right now. But I would really miss my flowers. I understand that they don't let you plant things in those retirement communities."

"Yes, I believe you can plant flowers around your condo."

"Well, I can't get out to work in the garden anymore anyway."

As I prepared to leave, he said: "It really makes me feel good to know that the church cares enough to send someone to keep me company. And I'm glad it's you."

After dinner that evening, I took Clarice to the mall to show her the necklace I wanted to give her for our anniversary. "They have a no-refund policy, so I want to make sure you like it."

She liked it.

On Sunday morning at church I bounced around, singing with one quartet, rehearsing with another, greeting people coming in from vacation. After church we planned to attend our neighborhood annual picnic, then go to an eagerly awaited outdoor concert.

Something changed when I stretched out for a short Sunday afternoon nap. Disturbing images began flashing into my mind. As I started to drift off, my subconscious would land me somewhere I did not want to go. My rational mind would cut it off and force me awake. It was as if I had walked into a movie theater, found that the movie was not to my liking, then walked out. I cycled through several of those episodes before finally sleeping.

I awoke dizzy and groggy. My eyes would not focus. Disturbing images swirled around my brain. I wanted to stay in my shell. I dreaded going to the picnic. But duty called. Clarice had fixed a casserole. I dragged myself out to eat hamburgers and exchange trivialities with neighbors. The conversation ranged through such critical subjects as plumbing and lawn maintenance problems.

Clarice and I had planned for several weeks to go to Symphony on the Prairie for an outdoor concert by the Preservation Hall Jazz Band, our all-time favorite jazz group. We had heard them at Preservation Hall, just off New Orleans' Bourbon Street. We had also heard them on concert tours. They always invigorated our spirits. Right now the greatest appeal was that it gave me an excuse to leave the picnic early.

We excused ourselves to drive out to the amphitheater on the grounds of Conner Prairie, a restored pioneer living-history park. I became so dizzy, I began stumbling. I started gasping for breath. I knew I was not in any condition to drive. "Do you want to stay home?" Clarice volunteered.

"I want to stay home. But I need to go." Sometimes I have to force myself to do what I know is good for me. I took half a Klonopin tablet and reminded myself to breathe slowly. By the time we arrived at Conner Prairie, my equilibrium was somewhat restored.

We faced light rain as we got out of the car. Armed with ponchos, lawn chairs, snacks, and a large umbrella, we found a spot to stake our claim on the grassy slope. Due to the threatening weather, the crowd was sparse. Maybe a thousand or so on a hillside that can accommodate six to ten thousand. The rain increased to a torrent.

Huddled in my lawn chair, under the umbrella, cocooned in my poncho, I felt depression beginning to clamp its vice around my head and chest. The rain eased up before concert time. As the musicians alternated intricate, soulful, and toe-tapping Dixieland, the vice eased its grip.

The band ended with their trademark "Just a Closer Walk with Thee," followed by "When the Saints Go Marching In." While playing "Saints," rain or no rain, they carried out their traditional parade through the audience. A couple hundred brave hearts poured out of their protective nests to march with them. With our jeans and feet drenched and our spirits refreshed, we headed home.

Monday morning. I had phone calls to make and errands to run before going to a back-to-school convocation downtown at the convention center. I couldn't wake up. My limbs would not move. Nor would my lips. I tried saying something to Clarice, but all that came out was an incoherent mumble. She did not try to rout me out of bed. She just kissed me good-bye and left for work.

Here I will let my journal speak.

[Journal, August 21, 2001] I try to force myself out of bed. I say to myself, "Try deep breathing—inhale for four counts. Hold for seven counts. Exhale for eight."

Myself answers, "Can't."

"Okay. Then try meditating." I find a pattern in the stuccoed ceiling plaster that looks like a dancing figure, and try to visualize myself as dancing.

Myself doesn't want to dance.

"Pray. Give thanks for life. Ask guidance for our children. Ask blessings on my beloved wife."

No good.

"Exercise! Stretch those arms! Arch your back! Lift your legs!"

Myself is becoming sarcastic. "Will clearing two inches satisfy you?"

I try to roll myself out of bed. Gravity takes over. I tell myself, "Just get up!"

Myself answers, "Myself is glued to the mattress. Can't move."

"That's stupid."

"So you say. Then you exert some effort and help push myself up."

I lie, panting for air, then doze off. Startled awake, I go through the whole process again. And again.

All the while I know what I really need to do. I tell myself: "Quit fighting. Don't try to force yourself. Completely relax, then roll over to the edge of the bed and onto your feet."

Myself answers, "You treat me like a child! You don't realize that my muscles are Jello."

> *I am poured out like water,*
>   *and all my bones are out of joint;*
> *my heart is like wax;*
>   *it is melted within my breast;*

my mouth is dried up like a potsherd,
and my tongue sticks to my jaws;
you lay me in the dust of death.[62]

It takes most of an hour to engage the simplest movement. Once on my feet, I drag myself, groaning all the way, to the bathroom to shave and dress.

I call Prince and take him out for a short walk. My feet are lead weights as I stagger up the slight incline to the woods path.

I don't think I can face breakfast. The thought of food is nauseating. I eat soda crackers and drink Pepsi to take my morning pills. I prepare to make phone calls. I begin stumbling and hyperventilating. The ghostly musical refrain that often accompanies my depressions oozes from the mildew in the back of my head: "O God, forgive my sins, I'm sick and old. O God, forgive my sins, I'm sick and old."[63]

When that refrain begins to haunt me, I counter with a chanted prayer, a mantra to chase away the demons of despair. The moment I stop my conscious chant, the ghost refrain seeps back in.

I begin gasping for air.

I begin sobbing.

I hear a long wail.

Where is it coming from? It is issuing from my own throat. I do not know it is emerging. Suddenly it is just—there. The wail continues unbroken for maybe half a minute.

Finally words break through: "O God, help me!"

I scold myself: "Keep busy! Keep busy! Don't give in!" I manage inconsequential tasks like collecting the trash and cleaning my moustache care kit. Another half hour and I am calm enough to place my phone calls. I call Clarice's office several times, just because I want to hear her voice. I get her voice mail each time.

I have planned to leave the house by eleven so I can get downtown, shop at Circle Center Mall, and eat lunch, before walking over to the convocation in the adjoining convention center. I finally crawl out of the house and into the car by 11:40. During the drive downtown, I begin to feel almost normal.

Conventioneers and shoppers choke the Circle Center food court. In the noise and crowd, I maintain composure long enough to order lunch and find a quiet table away from the food court in the Arts Garden.

From my table I can look out on the Washington Street traffic passing underneath the huge glass Arts Garden structure. I enjoy my Manchu Wok special number 3 while I read in Rachel Remen's book, *Kitchen Table Wisdom*.[64]

The convocation is scheduled for 1:00, so by 12:45 I head across the skybridge to the convention center. It is a three-block indoor walk to the assembly room. I start out in a brisk power-walk pace, but soon have to slow down due to the marauding hoards of teachers invading the convention center. If Indianapolis Public Schools do, indeed, have three thousand teachers, five thousand of them are trying to crowd through one entrance door.

I see no one I know.

I don't want to see anyone I know.

I want to be anonymous.

In the press and noise of the crowd,

I can feel the vice tightening down on my chest.

I begin gasping for breath.

I push back through the crowd and race into the huge hallway.

I find some water and take another half a Klonopin.

I lean against the wall, close my eyes, draw in slow breaths.

> *But you, O Lord, do not be far away!*
> *O my help, come quickly to my aid!*
> *Deliver my soul from the sword,*
> *my life from the power of the dog!*
> *Save me from the mouth of the lion!*[65]

Back in the assembly room, I stay on the edge of the crowd, trying to keep two or three body widths between myself and others. I know if I try to worm my way up the steep bleachers, I will have no escape. Looking down on the floor level, I see a few empty chairs. I take a chair on the second row, near enough to the side that I can get out if I have to.

I coerce myself to speak to the man sitting beside me. He pushes on me his agenda for what the school system should be doing. I try to listen. I am relieved when the superintendent stands to call the meeting to order. He never quite succeeds, but he starts anyway. As the speakers labor to cash in on their few minutes of public exposure, the crowd, still pushing through the door, creates a loud roar.

Speaker after speaker hammers on the theme of the day, which is the crying need for major capital improvements throughout the school system. As the convocation continues and the conversational roar from the back intensifies, I become more and more agitated. I decide that I will stay until 1:45, and then make a break for it. I keep my promise to myself.

Myself says, "What took you so long?"

I make it to the car and drive up to Fairview Church, where I have my private voice studio. I have an hour before my afternoon teaching schedule is to begin. I still feel foggy and dizzy when I arrive. I go to the youth lounge, find a comfortable recliner, and doze off. After thirty minutes I awake refreshed, energized, ready to face the day.

> *From the horns of the wild oxen*
> *you have rescued me.*
> *I will tell of your name to my*
> *brothers and sisters;*
> *in the midst of the congregation*
> *I will praise you.*[66]

This depression-anxiety cycle lasted twenty-five hours.

My Monday afternoon students are adults who have become good friends. We usually visit about as much as we sing. One of them, divorced with grandchildren, is so excited about her upcoming wedding that she can hardly sing at all.

I enjoy the teaching time, then head downtown again to meet a couple of friends at Charley and Barney's bar. We get together every couple of weeks, order soft drinks, and talk about things of importance to us. It is an informal outgrowth of relationships established through the Steven Ministry. Never before have I had a regular "night out with the boys." The more we meet, the more I realize how much these men and I have to share with one another.

I return home to my loving wife. It has been a rich day.

CHAPTER 40

THE BIG ONE

Tuesday, September 11, 2001. I am at home, working on my chronicle. Clarice calls. "I don't want to alarm you, but turn on the radio or television. Terrible things are happening all over." 8:46 AM. A Boeing 767 loaded with passengers had become a terrorist bomb, smashing into the World Trade Center in New York. I tuned in just after the second plane hit. My mind cannot fathom what my eyes are seeing. More is to come. Another Boeing, this one a 757, smashes into the Pentagon. A fourth crashes in Pennsylvania. This morning lives are changed as surely as they were on December 7, 1941, and on November 23, 1963.

With all air traffic halted, Joi, Joe, and their children, with Jon, are stranded on the southern tip of the Baja California peninsula, in Mexico, on what was supposed to be a business vacation.

Knowing that two of my children, both granddaughters, and my son-in-law are stuck, not knowing how they are to solve their dilemma, I arrive at Broad Ripple High School around 11:30. Classes are suspended. Students watch the unfolding cataclysm on the classroom TV monitors. They have been watching all morning. Many are numb, unable to comprehend an event so monumental. As I listen to the students talk, I realize that those young minds, unable to express the horrors seen, are allowing personal concerns to squeeze out through the cracks in their defenses.

I do no normal teaching this day. It was two hours before I even get to my studio.

A mother arrives at school to tell her daughter that the girl's father has died. The student, in a fit of impotent rage, beats up on her mother.

I learn that one of my students had been raped at knifepoint several weeks earlier. "We wanted you to know. But none of us wanted to be the one to tell you," another of my students explained.

I learn from a mother that her daughter, also my student, had engaged in self-mutilation and had made several suicide attempts.

I hear details of two divorces.

Tuesday progresses. We learn of more national horrors. We brace ourselves for what the next days might bring. Clarice is nearing her emotional limits. I want to be strong for her. I remember Rachel Remen's insistence that only the wounded can heal. Expertise can cure, but only compassion can heal. I catch myself coming down with a serious case of pride. *I am sick, so I can heal you.*

My rational mind tells me that I am in dangerous territory. I know that if I am going to invest myself emotionally in someone else, I must prepare for it. For the cataclysm of September 11, however, nobody is prepared. *God is my rock. I am not the rock. I am a millstone that I tie around my own neck.* Several times I feel myself buckling under the weight.

It would finally require a twenty-six-hour bus trip, with the two babies, zigzagging up the Baja California peninsula, to get Joi and her family, along with Jon, back to Tijuana and San Diego. During that trip they would have only one meal stop and one bathroom stop. They would be stopped several times at military checkpoints. We would not find out until Saturday that they were safely out of Mexico and home: Joi, Joe, and children to San Jose, Jon to Charlotte.

Prince, our twelve-year-old Labrador retriever, was full of cancer. We knew that his time was limited. On that Saturday morning after the attacks, I took Prince for a walk. I became nauseous trying to clean his infected ear. I caught myself thinking, *It would be so easy to choke him, say*

he dropped dead, and have a burial for him. He was so gentle, so loving, he would do anything to please me. I called him to me. He lumbered toward me, revealing the pain he was in. I threw my arms around his neck, scratched his back. I could never harm him. I wept, begging his forgiveness. I led him back to the house. Clarice came in. I kept my back to Clarice so she would not see my reddened eyes.

Sunday morning, September 16. With the millstone firmly locked to my neck, I do my duty and go to church. David's sermon tries to address our national healing and our national responsibilities. The millstone still hangs there.

At lunch Clarice and I decide we have to do something crazy. We go to the silliest movie we can find. *Rat Race* fills the bill. We laugh until our sides hurt.

Tears and laughter are twins.

A few days later, I had a dream in which that silly movie formed the framework. I was one of three teenage boys in a race, complete with obstacles and a final dash to a locker that held the prize, just like in the movie. The prizes included a trip to the Holy Land.

The whole competition was staged to test our character. Cooperation and compassion won out over aggression. I woke up singing "Dulcinea," from *Man of La Mancha.* Don Quixote, the mad knight errant of La Mancha, saw people not as they were, but as they could be.

The Premarin continued to work, bringing the PSA to 43.0 in November, down from 97.0 in May and 78.5 in July. A new CT scan showed that the swollen lymph nodes had shrunk by 50 percent. Yet the daily pressures of teaching at two locations created unrelenting fatigue. Rarely could I work a full day. I often cancelled or rearranged my schedule. Students and colleagues let me know that they were noticing my behavior.

After school, on a gray Thursday in December, I sat at the bar in Einstein's Bagels, sipping very hot Lemon Lift tea, chewing on a toasted plain bagel with honey-almond cream cheese, wondering where my spirits had gone. A wet, dreary day looked at me across the parking lot. A line of Paul Verlaine's played through my mental tapes: *Il pleure dans mon coeur comme il pleut dans la ville* (My heart weeps like the rain in the village).

Einstein's staff were all wearing Santa hats. "Auld Lang Syne" played on the Muzak. Cell phone calls around me jarred my head. I felt like a leaky tire. I kept pumping myself up, but as soon as I stopped pumping, I would deflate. I forced myself out to my Honda Civic and drove to my studio at Fairview to begin my afternoon teaching.

I stumbled, sobbing, into the building, choking out a simplistic prayer, certainly not worthy of literary or theological note. *Okay, God, here's the deal: You fix my leaks. You pump me up.*

The gasping and stumbling stopped.

My first student, a bright student from Cathedral High School, was waiting. We had a very productive voice lesson. Her mom and her three-year-old sister, Jessica, waited in the lounge. Jessica is the same age as Emily, my first grandchild. When I opened the studio door at the end of the lesson, Jessica came running down the hall, her arms wide, yelling "Skinny-cat! Skinny-cat!" When I had tried teaching Jessica this trick the previous week, she had not quite gotten the hang of it. Now she reached up and grabbed my hands. I picked her up. She tucked her knees, pulled up her feet, and pushed off from my stomach, somersaulting to the floor as I held her hands. A perfect skinny-cat. Jessica jumped up and down, clapping her hands, squealing, "I did it! I did it!"

Life is made of these moments.

Every Christmas I write a personal letter to each member of our family. As Christmas 2001 approached, I wrote to Clarice:

How to talk about love? We have survived another year and have come out stronger and closer. I can believe. I can surmise. I can guess. I can analyze. I can solve. But there are few things I know. I don't know how you love me. I don't even yet know all the subtle turns of your mind. I don't know how to bring world peace. I don't know how to bring harmony among friends.

But I do know this: Our love, rooted in the love of God, binds us, gives us independent life, and makes us strong. Every day, like a newborn child, our love is reborn. How can something mature be reborn? Perhaps like a rosebush that puts out new growth. Or a fallen maple tree that sprouts a new branch.

I don't know how. I just know.

CHAPTER 41

EUREKA

I n January 2002 a graduate student from Indiana University called
me. He was writing his doctoral dissertation on the vocal peda-
gogy of Herald "Prof" Stark, my teacher from the University of
Iowa. Would I be willing to let him interview me? Not only willing, I
promised him that he would feel like he had been with the Ancient
Mariner. The student came over. We sat in the living room. He turned on
his tape recorder, and we talked.

Reflecting on the interview afterward, I experienced several "eureka"
moments:

I remembered the gratitude I owe to Prof.

I realized how proud I am to have been his student.

At the time of the interview, I was the same age, sixty, that Prof was
when I began studying with him.

His own singing got better after he was sixty. Mine can, too.

By revisiting his teaching, I realized ways to improve my own
teaching.

Facing his professional activity that lasted until he was nearly ninety,
I realized that I still have much creative life left.

I no longer fear growing old.

This experience dovetailed with the book I was currently reading:

We are all here for but a single purpose:
to grow in wisdom
and to learn to love better.
We can do this by losing
as well as winning,
by having and by not having,
by succeeding or failing.
All we need to do
is show up openhearted
for class. . . .
You have to be present to win.[67]

I had not always been openhearted, or even present. Right after
reading that challenge by Rachel Remen, I recalled a painful experience of 1965. I had just finished my master's degree, and felt some desperation about getting a job. I spent the summer at a church assembly
on the Atlantic waterfront, working in the office and directing the staff
choir. Twin brothers, Jerry and Johnny, high school seniors, were the
best baritones in the choir. They were also lifeguards. Johnny was
handsome and easygoing. Jerry was homely and cynical. In a jest, I
compared Jerry unfavorably with his brother. His face clouded and his
eyes turned to fire.

"*Mister* Stegall—I am very aware of my own limitations."

I was mortified at what I had said, but was too proud to make
amends. I have no idea what happened to those young men or where
they might be. But my callousness at that moment has haunted me since
that time.

"Show up openhearted for class." That's tough. That's a risk. At age
twenty-four, I was not willing. And it still pains me.

Someone asked me, "Are those hormones changing your voice?"

"No, but I've caught myself singing 'I Enjoy Being a Girl.'"

February 2002 moved into March. Stress with work, friends, and family gnawed at me. I had been on the Premarin treatment for nearly a year. I was tired all the time. I could not maintain concentration. Food tasted bad. One of my students, after describing to me the tensions in her family over her choice of college, looked up at me with a little grin, and said, "I'm giving up stress for Lent." A few days later, when I could not function, I decided to try her suggestion. I skipped school. Eating lunch at Glendale Shopping Center food court, I threw up my lunch all over my tray.

Later in the spring my body got a chronic case of stubborn droops. Dr. Logan didn't think my Premarin treatments should have much to do with the excessively low energy. Neither did Dr. Shiller.

I checked back in with my primary physician. "Look, Jack, my oncologist and urologist don't think my treatments are a factor in my exhaustion."

"Baloney." That's an exact quote. With that sort of thing, I have total recall.

"So you think there may be a link between Premarin and exhaustion-nausea?"

"Bullseye!"

Add sextuple doses of hormones to cancer that would not go away. Factor in my autoimmunity. Factor in stresses of a school program heading for the rocks. Factor in traumas that members of my family were living through. Add it up: a good recipe for total disintegration.

I began taking yoga classes through the Wellness Community, a cancer education and support organization. As I got into yoga, I realized that the deep breathing and stretching I had been doing to prepare for singing all those years was all yoga. *Yoga* means unity of mind, body, and spirit.

During a sleepless night in April, a meditation on healing light generated itself:

Imagine light entering your body through your open hands.
The light absorbs into your skin and permeates your body.
Imagine that the light also reflects off your hands
like a pair of mirrors.

You can then direct the light in any direction you choose.
The healing light of Christ allows no shadows.
Wherever it shines becomes pure light.
Accept that light with gratitude.
Turn the "mirrors" of your palms toward you.
Where do you most need healing?
Move your hands in a slow circle
over the part of your body that represents your healing need.

At two o'clock in the morning, I am jolted wide awake, wrestling with a dilemma. When I pray for health, I am praying for destruction of sickness. At 2:00 AM. I puzzle over the two laws of thermodynamics.

The first law I learned in high school physics. Matter can be neither created nor destroyed. It can only change form. Matter may become energy or another form of matter. Combine two gasses, hydrogen and oxygen, and get a liquid, water, with totally different properties from either of the separate elements.

I did not learn the second law of thermodynamics in high school physics. Our class passed over it. The law of entropy. Every time matter changes form, a certain portion is lost to usefulness forever. When gas is used for heat, the heat cannot be recovered as gas. When medicine attacks and destroys sick cells, it also harms healthy cells.

My healing light imagery takes on a new, urgent focus: transform bad cells into good cells with a minimum of waste residue.

I move my hands over my lower abdomen.
I visualize the reflected healing light shining on cancerous lymph nodes.
I visualize the light shining on cancerous bone spots.
I can picture them easily.
I have seen their portraits on CT scans and bone scans.
I see the lymph nodes shrinking.
I see healthy bone marrow replacing destructive cells.
I see cancerous cells transforming into healthy bone marrow.

Now my rational brain hits an obstacle. It knows that one thing must die if another is to be born. My visualization becomes blurred. How do I get past it? Sometimes I see dead cancer cells being flushed out by natural processes. Do you transform or do you destroy? According to the law of entropy, both functions are inevitably present. Physical medicine seeks to destroy more than to transform. I take Premarin to destroy testosterone in order to starve cancer cells in order for healthy cells to grow unimpeded. The image of the healing light seeks not to destroy but to transform sick cells into healthy ones. The residue will pass harmlessly from the body through

breathing
sweating
urinating
defecating.
The healing light image goes further.
Turn your palms outward. Beams of healing light reflect off your palms
*   like mirrors. Do you see a person you know to be*
sick?
troubled?
in pain?
in mental darkness?
grieving?
Physically direct your light toward that person, and visualize that light
*   from Christ, reflected from your palms, shining outward to focus on*
*   that person's needs, transforming*
sickness into health,
injury into healing,
grieving into acceptance,
guilt into redemption.

The law of entropy warns us: Be prepared to lose something when you give. Jesus felt the power go out of him when the woman touched the hem of his garment. He spent much time in fasting and praying, to receive so that he could give. When we receive without giving, the gift shrivels. When we give without receiving, the reservoir dries up.

I remember John Shea's paradigm of the four most important words of healing: "Freely receive, freely give."

Freely receive.
Freely give.

✳

When I read through my 2001 journal in preparation for writing about events of that previous year, I told Clarice, "So much of the journal writing seems so dark."

Her response: "We had a lot of dark times last year."

In May I had a dream that I preferred not to talk about. I didn't want to talk about it because I didn't understand it. The clear message of the dream: *You are bombing the wrong target.* What could that mean? It would not explain itself.

I felt like my body was falling apart. Fatigue was becoming worse. I felt like my teaching efforts were half-hearted. I felt like I was cheating my students and making life tense for Clarice. I did not know what else to do, except to redouble my efforts. But was I doing the right things? Was I pushing a door that said, "Pull"?

My body kept telling me: *I can't keep going at the present pace.* It was time to do something new. I made a difficult decision. I applied for a medical leave from teaching.

In order to document the need for the leave, I had to emphasize the negatives. I had to tell what I can't do. I had to reveal the medical certainty that I had advancing cancer.

The prospect presented the dilemma: If I am to allow my body the rest and the relief from stress that is necessary for healing, I must admit, officially, to being sick.

I have to keep reminding myself that accepting a diagnosis does not enslave me to a prognosis.

Early in the summer, my younger son asked, "Dad, what are you doing this summer?"

I instantly decided: "Writing and getting my book published. That's my job right now."

"Pays about as good as music, doesn't it?"

The 2002 ADM music conference was held in July in Oklahoma City. Because Clarice and I had not attended for two years, we wondered how many of "that old gang of ours" would attend. To our great satisfaction, it was a rich homecoming. We shared a full week of music, worship, visiting, and affirmation. I called Arthur Smith, our friend from my previous school. After being a widower for seven years, he had remarried in 2000. On our free afternoon, he drove up to Oklahoma City, introduced us to his delightful bride, took us out for lunch and to visit the Oklahoma City National Memorial.

When we returned home to Indianapolis, on top of the accumulated mail was a letter from the school board. What would it say? By requesting medical leave, I felt like I was giving up. Yet I really did not think that I could face another year of the pace and stress that had been so much a part of my multitasking life.

I read the letter. Relief. A semester off with pay. Good deal. Then another reality hit: For the first time since 1947, I was not gearing up for a school year. I had always been in school as a student or a teacher.

In August 2002 a new bone scan did not detect any bone spots. The area where the spots had been was now clear. A new CT scan showed shrinkage of the lymph nodes. My PSA was down to 21.0, after spiking at 92.0 in April.

The story continues. The disease takes on new forms. For prostate cancer, chemotherapy is way down at the end of the list of treatments. Through surgery, radiation, two forms of hormone treatment—then chemotherapy—I'm still here. After surviving the first three years, I consider that I am living on "free" time. Every day is a gift of grace. I am grateful for every chance to tell Clarice I love her, to play with the grandchildren, to visit my children, to go out with friends.

Though I live mindful of the past and hopeful for the future, I have only the moment. In *The Music Man*, Harold Hill says to Marian Paroo: "My dear little librarian—Pile up enough tomorrows and you'll find you've collected nothing but a lot of empty yesterdays. I don't know about you, but I'd like to make today worth remembering."[68]

Samuel F. Pugh is a retired Disciples of Christ minister and retired editor of the Disciples' national magazine. While I was minister of music at Downey Avenue Christian Church, Sam was a constant inspiration to me. Already a man of tiny stature, he physically shrank as arthritis ate away his knees and his hips. Sam is one of the most loving, accepting people I have ever known. He once brought me several of his poems; then we collaborated in writing a hymn.

In December 1999 the *Indianapolis Star* printed a story on people who had witnessed the changes of the twentieth century. The account featured Sam. In the interview he observed that the flush toilet had made a greater impact on civilization than had the airplane! Another news story in 2001 showed Sam, at age ninety-seven, volunteering at a preschool.

In 1952 Sam wrote "For a Day of My Life," which was widely circulated as "Anonymous" for a number of years. He has given me blanket permission to use his thoughts:

> This is the beginning of a new day.
> God has given me this day to use as I will.
> I can waste it, or use it for good, but what I do today is important
> because I am exchanging a day of my life for it.
> When tomorrow comes this day will be gone forever,
> leaving behind in its place something that I have traded for it.
> I want it to be gain and not loss, good and not evil,
> success and not failure, in order that I shall not regret
> the price that I have paid for it.[69]

APPENDIX

SO YOU WANT
JUST THE FACTS?

A User's Guide to Prostate Cancer (with a few opinions thrown in)

First, what's the bad news?
Nearly 190,000 new cases of prostate cancer show up in the United States each year. Over 30,000 men will die of the disease this year. If you wait until you feel symptoms, it may be too late.

Is there any good news?
Yes. There is plenty of good news. The American Cancer Society reports, "Eighty-three percent of all prostate cancers are discovered in the local and regional stages; the five-year relative survival rate for patients whose tumors are diagnosed at these stages is 100 percent. Over the past twenty years, the survival rate for all stages combined has increased from 67 percent to 96 percent."[70] The increase in survival is due largely to early detection and treatment, made possible by the development of the PSA test. This test has been the primary early detection tool since 1988.

That's enough statistics. Where do I fit in?
Are you over fifty years of age? Get your PSA tested every year. If you have a family history of prostate cancer, start tests at forty. If you are

African American, you should be tested by age forty, because you are at a slightly higher risk than are European Americans.

You keep saying "PSA"—What is it?

PSA (Prostate Specific Antigen) is a form of enzyme, a protein that regulates the rate of a chemical reaction in the body. Once thought to be inert, PSA has been shown to turn viscous semen into liquid after it leaves the body, making it possible for the sperm to swim up into the uterus.

Where is PSA produced?

PSA is produced primarily by the prostate gland. It is also produced by prostate cancer. It occurs in trace amounts in other organs, in breast cancer cells, and in the salivary glands and adrenal glands.

Don't those trace amounts compromise the PSA as a marker for cancer?

No. One gram of cancer tissue produces ten times the amount of PSA as does one gram of normal tissue.

How do I get my PSA checked?

PSA level can be checked by a blood test. Many physicians routinely order it as part of an annual checkup.

What is a normal level?

Most physicians consider a safe PSA level to be 4.0 nanograms per milliliter of serum (ng/ml). New evidence suggests a lower "safe" threshold."[71] Many men produce a high PSA and are free of disease. According to Patrick Walsh, MD, "Only 25 percent of men with a PSA between 4 and 10 will turn out to have cancer."[72] After prostatectomy (surgical removal of the prostate), under 1.0 ng/ml is considered safe.

Then what does an elevated PSA mean?

It can mean that the gland is either
  (1) enlarged
  (2) infected
  (3) cancerous

It may, in rare instances, indicate abnormalities in other organs. If you show a high reading, follow-up tests and examinations are needed to determine the cause.

What about the noncancerous causes of high PSA?
BPH (Benign Prostatic Hyperplasia), also called **BHP** (Benign Hyperplasic Prostate), is a nondiseased, enlarged prostate. It may produce a high PSA reading. If the swollen gland interferes with urination, the goal is to shrink it, usually through herbal or hormonal treatment. On rare occasions it may be necessary to core it out surgically (transurethral resection), or to remove the entire prostate gland.

Prostatitis is an infection of the prostate. It, too, may produce an elevated PSA. For that reason, if there has been a previously elevated PSA reading, the urologist may prescribe an antibiotic prior to taking a follow-up PSA.

What if the PSA continues to be high?
If you are already taking an annual PSA test, keep tabs on changes in the reading. A high reading that remains stable is cause for caution and watchful waiting. A steady rise in PSA is the main clue indicating cancer.

What's with the latex glove?
DRE (digital rectal exam) involves the physician inserting his finger into the rectum to determine prostate abnormalities. The prostate gland is just anterior to the rectum, so its surface can be felt by pressure on the rectal wall.[73]

But what does the DRE tell you?
The DRE can tell your doctor about abnormalities, hardening, or unusual size of the prostate. Since abnormalities may not be malignant, the DRE by itself is not a definitive cancer diagnosis tool. It is, though, an essential part of the diagnosis process. Until around 1988, the DRE was the only early detection method.

Where does the needle come in?
Biopsy is the sampling of tissue to check for malignancy. For a prostate biopsy, the urologist inserts a probe into the rectum. Guided by ultrasound imagery, the urologist uses the instrument to insert a needle through the rectal wall and into the prostate gland (it's just anterior to the rectum). The usual biopsy takes six or more needle core samples in a matter of a few minutes. You may feel the stings. You may feel pressure. You may feel nothing. Even six to ten needle samples may miss a tiny cancer.

What about aftereffects from the biopsy?
It may be prudent to abstain from sex for a few days, because blood may show up in urine, feces, and semen.

That means that diagnosis is a three-step process?
Yes. You need all three: PSA test, DRE, and biopsy.

I hear about a "stage B-1" cancer. What does that mean?
There are several measuring systems. Your physician may use one or more of these. **Stages** are most commonly measured by letters:
A: microscopic
B1: detectable as a lump during DRE, and confined to one side
B2: more than two cm in diameter, or on both sides of the gland
C: spread throughout the prostate
Positive margin: malignant cells on the outside of the gland
D1: malignancy spread to surrounding tissues
D2: malignancy spread (metastasized) to other organs or the bones

Gleason score is a measure of the degree of malignancy within the prostate. It uses a scale of 1 to 10.
1: well-differentiated, looking much like a normal gland
5: moderately differentiated, moderately invasive
10: poorly differentiated, most intrusive, most aggressive

TNM grading system:
T: measures size of **tumor**
N: measures metastasis (spreading) to lymph **nodes**
M: measures **metastasis** to other parts of the body

Differentiation? Please explain.
Differentiation refers to variations in the appearance of prostate cancer cells. Well-differentiated cells are clearly defined, uniform in shape and distribution. Poorly differentiated cells are of abnormal shape and are clumped together to form tumor masses.

Uh-oh. My biopsy shows cancerous tissue in the prostate. Now what?
Prostate cancer is slow growing. If you are over seventy-five years of age and are just discovering an early-stage cancer, you may not need any treatment.

If you have an enlarged prostate, you may need therapy to shrink it before going ahead with other treatments. Herbal treatments such as PC-SPES, steroids such as prednisone, or hormone treatments such as Lupron will shrink swollen tissue and may bring down the PSA. We do not yet have strong evidence that these procedures actually reduce cancer.

First-line treatments of prostate cancer may take several forms:
- Radioactive seed implantation (brachytherapy) may be a good choice if the cancer is in very early stages. Brachytherapy is constantly being refined so that it can pinpoint exact spots.
- Freezing the cancer with liquid nitrogen (cryosurgery), which fell out of use due to the greater accuracy and success of brachytherapy. As of 2001, there were no long-term randomized multicenter tests, so the long-term effectiveness has not been proven.[74]
- Surgery to remove the prostate (radical prostatectomy), is a good choice if tests show the cancer to be contained within the prostate. A catch: if stage and aggressiveness is uncertain, surgery is the only way to see, for sure, whether there is any positive margin (cancer cells on the outer wall of the prostate), or any spreading beyond the gland.
- External beam radiation may be used alone, or as a follow-up to surgery. You can have surgery before radiation, but it doesn't work to do radiation before surgery.

Will surgery and/or radiation clear it up?
Surgery or radiation will clear the cancer in 80 to 85 percent of the cases that are caught early. The American Cancer Society affirms a 100 percent five-year survival rate for persons who get early detection and early treatment.

You haven't said anything about chemotherapy. Is it effective?
Chemotherapy is not an effective first- or second-line treatment for prostate cancer. It may come into play later used in combination with other forms of treatment.

What about impotence?
Different treatments carry varying risks of impotence.
- Seed implantation and cryosurgergy have the best odds against impotence.

- Radiation causes less impotence than surgery.
- Surgery carries the greatest risk of impotence.
- "Nerve-sparing" surgery lowers the impotency risk.

If I become impotent, then what?

Even here, you have cause for encouragement.

- Nerve-sparing surgery, which preserves some of the erectile nerves on the surface of the prostate gland, may allow erection and a "dry" orgasm. This procedure can be used only when the tumor is totally contained within the gland, and if there is no positive margin.
- Sexual stimulation and orgasm may be possible without erection.
- As procedures become more refined, the chances of maintaining some potency keep getting better.

Will Viagra do any good?

If the erectile nerves are at least partially intact after surgery, Viagra can give them a boost. It does not increase the sex drive or the ability to reach orgasm.

But what if those nerves are taken out?

Several mechanical aids are on the market, including vacuum pumps and implants. Mechanical aids do not produce sexual feeling.

Will surgery make me incontinent?

Possibly. The urethra, which carries urine from the bladder to the penis, has three pairs of sphincter muscles that serve as check valves for urine flow. The prostate gland wraps around the urethra and the middle of those three pairs of muscles.

- The top pair, at the base of the bladder, may be taken out or damaged.
- Surgery removes part of the urethra, including the middle pair.
- The third, lowest, pair will be kept open during the time you have a catheter. Muscle function may atrophy during that time.

Is bowel function a factor?

In some cases:

- Surgery may damage bowel control nerves.
- Radiation can damage the rectum, becoming a factor in bowel incontinence.

Can one repair the damage?
Simple exercises can improve muscle tone to the point that incontinence may become a minor factor, or may clear it up completely.

Then why have the surgery to start with?
It may not be right for you, or it may be the only sure treatment.

What does it mean if the PSA stays high after treatment?
A continued elevated PSA reading after surgery and radiation often indicates that the cancer has spread elsewhere. You may have elevated or fluctuating PSA levels but no physical symptoms. In that case your next move would be to bring the PSA down and be alert for symptoms, such as swollen lymph nodes or bone spots.

What do we do if the PSA won't come down?
The usual next step is to shut off the testosterone stimulation of cancer growth through hormone therapy or orchiectomy.

How does hormone therapy work?
Hormone treatment either counteracts or shuts off testosterone. Testosterone, along with other androgens (male hormones), especially dihydrotestosterone, is the main growth stimulant for prostate cancer. Several forms of hormone treatment are available. Those derived from estrogen, the female hormone, counteract or neutralize the effects of testosterone. Other products actually shut off the testosterone production. The most common current treatment is Lupron, administered by injection either once a month or once every three months. Casodex, a daily pill, is often used as a supplement to the Lupron.

Bilateral orchiectomy—is that what I think it is?
Yes. Surgical removal of the testicles is another means of shutting down 90 percent of androgen (male hormone) production, including testosterone. The effects are similar to hormone treatment. Orchiectomy is surgical castration. Hormone blockage is medical castration.

Am I then treatment-free?
Probably not. The adrenal glands account for about 10 percent of the androgen production. Orchiectomy and Lupron will not affect this

production. A supplemental drug such as Casodex will help block testosterone production from the adrenals and other places.

Okay—We've pulled out the artillery, and it won't go away. Now what?
The most common places for prostate cancer to settle are the lymph glands and the bones. When it attaches to another part of the body, it is still prostate cancer. Spot radiation may shrink swollen tissues and relieve pain, but it is not a cure. Cancer has a mind of its own. Eventually it can find something other than testosterone to allow it to grow. In that case it will become active again, and the hormone treatment will no longer be effective. In the event that the cancer becomes impervious to hormones, combinations of chemotherapy and other treatments are showing some promise.

Aren't there other ways to kill off the bad cells?
As of yet we don't have proven ways to destroy the cancer once it has spread. We do have some inhibiting treatments that can slow down the growth.

Antiangiogenesis[75] agents inhibit the formation of new blood vessels. To grow, a tumor must generate blood vessels to supply it with food. An antiangiogenesis agent would stop the original tumor growth, and it would inhibit the spread of cancer to the bones, liver, and other tissues. These agents are experimental, and their effectiveness has been disappointing[76] because there are many angiogenic (blood-vessel-forming) factors that must be blocked.

Prednisone and other steriods can shrink swollen tissues and increase feelings of well being. They may bring down the PSA. As long as the PSA remains stable or comes down, there will likely not be further advancement of the cancer.

Premarin and other estrogen extracts can shrink swollen tissues and bone spots. They can also strengthen the bones, making them more resistant to cancerous growth.

Do I hear some more bad news on its way?
It can be. Once the cancer has spread, we work for containment and relief of discomfort. We do not yet have a cure. Radiation can clear out specific "hot spots" of malignancy in the bones. It can shrink swollen tissues. New combinations of hormonal, herbal, steroidal, and chemo therapy can bring relief from discomfort. Even so, at that point cancer has developed

a life of its own. Treatment may not prolong your life. It can, however, make your life better.

So—prostate cancer kills, right?
Not necessarily, and increasingly rarely. Prostate cancer grows very slowly. Almost every man who gets early detection and treatment is still alive five years later. If you discover cancer after you are seventy-five, you might outlive it with no treatment.

Are those treatments the only game in town?
Not at all. You have many options, such as special diets, exercise, herbal treatments, meditation, and prayer. Such practices boost your overall health and rally your own immune system. They are good for you, whether you are healthy or sick.

Can following a health regimen replace medical treatment?
The jury is still out on that question. There are too many unknowns, too few studies, and too many risks to forgo medical treatment in favor of alternatives. Many physicians, however, view alternative treatments as allies to medical treatment.

I keep getting contradicting opinions. How do I filter them out?
• Seek out the most reliable information you can get.[77]
• Find a prostate cancer specialist who is open to all forms of treatment.
• Read the fine print. Know what possible side effects a treatment may carry.
• Learn about nontraditional treatments if you choose.
• Realize that your belief system is going to have a powerful influence on your choices.
• Talk with your physicians, counselors, support group, family, and friends.
• Finally, you are the boss. You choose your own treatment.

But I'm the backbone for my family. I don't want to worry them.
You don't want to worry them? Then engage your family in your quest. Keeping your concerns to yourself does not protect them. Your spouse may wind up having to take depression treatment so she can put up with

you. Take your spouse, partner, or a trusted friend with you to appointments, particularly if you are advancing to a new level of treatment. Another set of ears can help you in making your decisions. *A strong, open relationship with your loved ones is the most important force in their well being and in your healing.*

I still have a lot of questions. Where can I go?
The bibliography of this book can point you to many sources. These two deserve special attention:

Sheldon Marks, MD, urologist, prostate cancer specialist, has written an excellent, thorough book, *Prostate and Cancer: A Family Guide to Diagnosis, Treatment, and Survival* (Fisher Books, 1995, 1997, 1999, 2001). As of this writing, a new edition is in the works. Marks covers everything, beginning with a healthy prostate to describing and diagramming all stages of prostate disease, diet, treatments, recovery, and what one can expect when treatment fails.

Patrick C. Walsh, MD, professor of urology at the Johns Hopkins Medical Institutions, is the surgeon who developed the nerve-sparing surgery. I have referred to his findings earlier in the body of the text and in this appendix. Using layman's language, his book details and diagrams all aspects of men's reproductive health. It is a superb tool for in-depth research of particular questions. It is not a good "first primer." He includes so much detail that it can be overwhelming to one who is just coming to grips with the disease.

BIBLIOGRAPHY

Sources marked with (*) are especially useful for basic information.
Sources marked with (+) focus on alternative healing.

Albertson, Peter C., MD. "Competing Risk Analysis of Men Aged 55 to 74 Years at Diagnosis Managed Conservatively for Clinically Localized Prostate Cancer," *Journal of the American Medical Association (JAMA)*, September 16, 1998, vol. 180, no. 11, 975.

Albom, Mitch. *Tuesdays with Morrie: An Old Man, a Young Man, and Life's Greatest Lesson.* New York: Doubleday, 1997.

* American Cancer Society. *Cancer Facts and Figures 2002,* updated annually.

Andersen, Hans Christian. "The Snow Queen," in *The Complete Hans Christian Andersen Fairy Tales*, edited by Lily Owens. New York: Crown Publishers, 1984.

+ Barraclough, Jennifer. *Cancer and Emotion: A Practical Guide to Psycho-oncology.* Hoboken, N. J.: John Wiley and Sons, 1994.

+ Cousins, Norman. *Anatomy of an Illness as Perceived by the Patient: Reflections on Healing and Regeneration.* New York: W. W. Norton, 1979.

+ _____. *Head First: The Biology of Hope.* San Francisco: E. P. Dutton, 1989.

D'Amico, Anthony V., MD, PhD, et al. "Biochemical Outcome after Radical Prostatectomy, External Beam Radiation Therapy, or

Interstitial Radiation Therapy for Clinically Localized Prostate Cancer," *JAMA,* September 16, 1998, vol 280, no.11, 969-980.

+ De Salvo, Louise, PhD. *Writing As a Way of Healing: How Telling Our Stories Transforms Our Lives.* San Francisco: HarperSanFrancisco, 1999.

+ Dossey, Larry, MD. *Be Careful What You Pray For . . . You Just Might Get It: What We Can Do about the Unintentional Effects of Our Thoughts, Prayers, and Wishes.* San Francisco: HarperSanFrancisco 1997.

+ _____. *Prayer Is Good Medicine.* San Francisco: HarperSanFrancisco, 1996.

+ _____. *Reinventing Medicine: Beyond Mind-Body to a New Era of Healing.* San Francisco: HarperSanFrancisco, 1996.

Enzler, Clarence. *Everyman's Way of the Cross.* Notre Dame, Ind.: Ave Maria Press, 1970, 1984.

+ Gardiner, Eric. *How I Conquered Cancer: A Naturopathic Alternative.* Houston: Emerald Ink Publishing, 1997.

* Garnick, Marc B., MD. *The Patient's Guide to Prostate Cancer: An Expert's Successful Treatment Strategies and Options.* New York: Plume Books, 1996.

Gomella, Leonard G., MD, and John J. Fried. *Recovering from Prostate Cancer.* New York: HarperBooks, 1993.

+ Hirshberg, Caryle and Marc Ian Barash. *Remarkable Recovery: What Extraordinary Healings Tell Us about Getting Well and Staying Well.* New York: Riverhead Books, 1995.

Holy Bible: New Revised Standard Version. Grand Rapids, Mich.: Zondervan Bible Publishers, 1989.

Kafka, Franz. *The Trial.* Translated and with a preface by Brean Mitchell. New York: Schocken Books, 1990, 1998. Originally published in German as *Der Prozess.* Berlin: Verlag die Schmiede, 1925.

* Kaltenbach, Don, with Tim Richards. *Prostate Cancer: A Survivor's Guide.* Sarasota, Fl.: Seneca House Press, 1996.

Korda, Michael. *Man to Man: Surviving Prostate Cancer.* New York: Random House, 1996.

* Loo, Marcus H., MD, and Marian Betancourt. *The Prostate Cancer Sourcebook: How to Make Informed Treatment Choices.* Hoboken, N. J.: John Wiley and Sons, 1998.

* Maddox, Robert L. *Prostate Cancer: What I Found Out and What You Should Know.* Phoenix, Az.: Harold Shaw Publishers, 1997.

* Marks, Sheldon, MD. *Prostate and Cancer: A Family Guide to Diagnosis, Treatment, and Survival.* Tuscon, Az.: Fisher Books, 1995, 1997, 1999, 2001 (new edition in the works).

McCarthy, Joe (lyrics), and James V. Monaco (music). "You Made Me Love You (I Didn't Want to Do It)." Broadway Music Corp., 1913.

Middlebrook, Christina, PhD. *Seeing the Crab: A Memoir of Dying.* New York: Basic Books, 1996.

* Morganstern, Stephen, MD, and Allen Abrahams, PhD. *The Prostate Sourcebook.* New York: Contemporary Books, 1993.

+ Moyers, Bill. *Healing and the Mind.* New York: Doubleday, 1993.

+ Nouwen, Henri J. M. *The Wounded Healer.* New York: Doubleday, 1972. Reprinted by Image Books, Doubleday, 1979.

* Oesterling, Joseph E., MD, and Mark A. Moyad, MPH. *The ABC's of Prostate Cancer: The Book That Could Save Your Life.* Lanham, Md.: Madison Books, 1997.

Price, Reynolds. *A Whole New Life: An Illness and a Healing.* New York: Atheneum/Macmillan Publishing Company, 1994.

Remen, Rachel Naomi, MD. *Kitchen Table Wisdom: Stories That Heal.* New York: Riverhead Books, 1996.

Scher, Howard I., MD. "Management of Prostate Cancer after Prostatectomy: Treating the Patient, Not the PSA," *JAMA,* May 5, 1999, vol. 281, no. 17, 1642-1645.

Shea, John. *Gospel Light: Jesus Stories for Spiritual Consciousness.* New York: Crossroad/Herder & Herder, 1998.

Shipley, et al. "Radiation Therapy for Clinically Localized Prostate Cancer: A Multi-Institutional Pooled Analysis," *JAMA,* May 5, 1999, vol. 281, no. 17, 1598.

+ Siegel, Bernie S., MD. *Love, Medicine, and Miracles: Lessons Learned about Self-Healing from a Surgeon's Experience with Exceptional Patients.* New York: Harper and Row, 1990.

+ _____. *Prescriptions for Living: Inspirational Lessons for a Joyful, Loving Life.* New York: HarperCollins, 1998.

* Simon, David, MD. *Return to Wholeness: Embracing Body, Mind, and Spirit in the Face of Cancer.* Hoboken, N. J.: John Wiley and Sons, 1999.

Smyth, Joshua, PhD, et al. "Effects of Writing about Stressful Experiences on Symptom Reduction in Patients with Asthma or Rheumatoid Arthritis: A Randomized Trial," *JAMA*, April 12, 1999, vol. 281, no. 14, 1304-1329.

Trillin, Alice. *Dear Bruno.* New York: The New Press, 1996.

* Wainrib, Barbara, and Sandra Haber. *Prostate Cancer: A Guide for Women and the Men They Love.* New York: Dell, 1996.

+ Wakefield, Dan. *Expect a Miracle.* San Francisco: HarperSanFrancisco, 1995.

* Walsh, Patrick C., MD, and Janet Farrar Worthington. *Dr. Patrick Walsh's Guide to Surviving Prostate Cancer.* New York: Warner Books, 2001.

+ Weil, Andrew, MD. *Spontaneous Healing: How to Discover and Enhance Your Body's Natural Ability to Maintain and Heal Itself.* New York: Ballantine, 1995.

+ _____. *Eight Weeks to Optimum Health: A Proven Program for Taking Full Advantage of Your Body's Natural Healing Power.* New York: Alfred A. Knopf, 1997.

Wilson, Meredith. *The Music Man.* New York: Music Theater International, 1950.

END NOTES

1. See appendix, "So You Want Just the Facts?"
2. This recent information came from Philip Snodgrass, MD, and was verified by Bruce Roth, MD.
3. In music, a 6/4 chord is the incomplete chord that precedes a complete cadence.
4. More recent studies verify Dr. Shiller's findings. Shipley et al.,"Radiation Therapy for Clinically Localized Prostate Cancer" *JAMA,* May 5, 1999, vol. 281, no. 17, 1598ff., shows that using radiation only for T1 and T2 tumors with a PSA of 10 or less and a Gleason score of 6 or less is about as effective as radical prostatectomy in preventing reoccurrence after five years. This article also identifies 1988 as the year the PSA began to be used as a marker of prostate cancer ("T1," etc., is a system for measuring the size of cancer that is contained within the prostate. My doctors used the more common A, B, C, D rating as explained in the appendix). "Gleason score" is a measure of the aggressiveness of the cancer (1: barely detectable. 10: fills the organ). My cancer would not have been a candidate for first-line radiation because I had a PSA of 37.1, a "C" rating, and a Gleason score of 7.
5. See commentary on D'Amico et al.
6. Five years later the procedure had been refined to make it more precise. In the celebrated case of South African Anglican Archbishop

Desmond Tutu (2000), cryosurgery was used as a follow-up to radiation. As of 2001, long-term effectiveness of cryosurgery (or cryo-oblation) was still not proven.

7. The appendix describes other uses of hormone therapy.
8. The nerve-sparing procedure, developed by Dr. Patrick Walsh of the Johns Hopkins Hospital in Baltimore, is now practiced routinely.
9. Garrison Keillor, *A Prairie Home Companion* (radio show).
10. Hans Christian Anderson, "The Snow Princess," published as "The Snow Queen" in *The Complete Hans Christian Anderson Fairy Tales*, ed. Lily Owens (New York: Crown Publishers, 1984), 53-73.
11. R. Carroll Stegall. May 18, 1989.
12. There are three sphincter muscles that serve as check valves for the urethra. The upper, involuntary, muscle is at the base of the bladder. The middle, also involuntary, muscle is within the prostate gland. The lower, voluntary, muscle is at the base of the urethra. During surgery the surgeon cuts away the top muscle and repositions it, causing damage so that it may or may not regain function. The middle muscle is removed. The lower muscle remains intact, but the catheter tube keeps it from closing. When the tube is removed, that muscle has to learn to function all over again. Removal of one muscle, damage to another, and atrophying of the third is the source of the urinary incontinence most men experience. I would much later learn of yet another complication: the surgery can damage nerves that trigger the sphincter muscle at the base of the colon, causing bowel incontinence.
13. From an Ann Landers column, published in *Indianapolis Star,* Thursday, June 29, 1995. Creators Syndicate, PO Box 11562, Chicago, IL 60611-0562.
14. DES was taken off the market in July 1997.
15. 1 Samuel, chapter 3.
16. "Sody Salaraytus" is widely published in many folktale sources. It became a signature piece for folktale pioneer Jackie Torrence. All tellers of folktales put their own stamps on the stories. My version is based on the first telling I heard of it, by my colleague David Titus.
17. Leonard G. Gomella, MD, and John J. Fried, *Recovering from Prostate Cancer* (New York: HarperPaperBacks, 1993), 95.
18. Yes! They all alliterate, as well as Clarice and Carroll, Lyle (her

brother) and Linda, and Joel (my brother) and June. Jeremy swears he will never marry a woman who alliterates.

19. Traditional Shaker song, "Simple Gifts."

20. Sabing Baring-Gould, "Onward, Christian Soldiers."

21. African American spiritual.

22. Luke 22:42.

23. And, later, also our granddaughters.

24. John 14:2.

25. For the purist who must know, it was J. S. Bach's Cantata no. 4, *Christ lag in Todesbanden* ("Christ Lay in Dead's Dark Prison").

26. Saul Alinksky, quoted in Peter McWilliams, *The Portable Do It!* (Santa Monica, Calif.: Prelude Press, 1995), 165.

27. Matthew 5:45.

28. Franz Kafka, *The Trial.* Translated and with a preface by Bream Mitchell (New York: Schocker Books, 1990, 1998). Originally published in German as *Der Prozess* (Berlin: Verlag die Schmiede, 1925).

29. "Indiana Today" ran for eleven years until it closed on Dec. 24, 2002.

30. John Shea, *Gospel Light: Jesus Stories for Spiritual Consciousness* (New York: Crossroad, 1998).

31. Susan Silberstein, quoted in Caryle Hirshberg and Marc Ian Barasch, *Remarkable Recovery* (New York: Riverhead Books, 1995), 302.

32. Louise de Salvo, *Writing As a Way of Healing: How Telling Our Stories Transforms Our Lives* (San Francisco: HarperSanFrancisco, 1999).

33. Joshua Smyth, PhD, et al., "Effects of Writing about Stressful Experiences on Symptom Reduction in Patients with Asthma or Rheumatoid Arthritis: A Randomized Trial," *JAMA,* April 12, 1999, vol. 281, no. 14, 1304-1329.

34. Joshua Smyth and Louise de Salvo on *The Diane Rehm Show,* WAMU, National Public Radio, May 5, 1999.

35. Henri Nouwen, *The Wounded Healer* (New York: Image Books, Doubleday, 1979), 38 (passage edited to be gender inclusive). Copyright 1972 by Henri J. M. Nouwen.

36. Research in prostate cancer is multiplying. As of this writing, over 125 trials are being conducted around the United States alone. We still don't have answers.

37. Bruce Roth, MD, moderating the monthly meeting of "The Common Bond," a prostate cancer support group, on October 21, 1997.

38. Howard I. Scher, MD, "Management of Prostate Cancer After Prostatectomy: Treating the Patient, Not the PSA," *JAMA*, May 5, 1999, vol. 281, no. 17, 1642–1645. Study by Pound et al. in same issue, 1591.

39. Anthony V. D'Amico, MD, PhD, et al., "Biochemical Outcome After Radical Prostatectomy, External Beam Radiation Therapy of Interstitial Radiation Therapy for Clinically Localized Prostate Cancer," *JAMA*, September 16, 1998, vol. 280, no. 11, 980. Responses to this study are printed in *JAMA*, May 5, 1999, vol. 281, no. 17, 1583-1586.

40. Romans 8:38-39.

41. Christina Middlebrook, *Seeing the Crab: A Memoir of Dying* (New York: HarperCollins BasicBooks, 1996), 4-5.

42. Mitch Albom, *Tuesdays with Morrie: An Old Man, A Young Man, and Life's Greatest Lesson* (New York: Doubleday, 1997), 104.

43. Marcus Borg, *Meeting Jesus Again for the First Time: The Historical Jesus and the Heart of Contemporary Faith* (San Francisco: HarperSanFrancisco, 1994).

44. I learned this mode of meditation in 1998, with Dr. Craig Overmyer, in Zionsville, Indiana. He summarizes his approach in his article "Waiting . . . patiently . . ." in *Healthy Living*, November 1999, 16.

45. John 9:25.

46. Joe McCarthy (lyrics) and James V. Monaco (music), "You Made Me Love You (I Didn't Want to Do it)" (Broadway Music Corporation, 1913).

47. Dream of being left behind, January 24, 1997, in chapter 22.

48. From my journal of November 18, 1999.

49. Gian-Carlo Menotti, *The Medium*, opera in one act (G. Schirmer, Inc.).

50. He did not change his name. He did go to a prestigious university, where he majored in music, became the first African American to be elected homecoming king, sang Escamillo in *Carmen*, finished his degree, and went on to take graduate studies in jazz, the first vocal jazz major at that school.

51. This sermon was given in 2000.

52. Aaron Copland, *Old American Songs, Part 2* (New York: Boosey and Hawkes, 1960).

53. Wake Forest College was soon renamed Wake Forest University.

54. Marcus Borg, *Meeting Jesus Again for the First Time* (San Francisco: HarperSanFrancisco, 1994), 13.

55. Attributed to George Croly, 1780–1860.

56. Clarence Enzler, *Everyman's Way of the Cross* (Notre Dame, Ind.: Ave Maria Press, 1970) 1984.

57. If you must know, or even if you don't care, I can vocalize from a bass low F to a soprano high C. My "good" singing range is from bass G to tenor A-flat.

58. A folk paraphrase of *Julius Caesar*, act 2, scene 2. Shakespeare wrote: "Cowards die many times before their deaths; the valiant never taste of death but once."

59. Anonymous, "Just a Closer Walk with Thee," often attributed to Thomas A. Dorsey.

60. Joe, my pharmacologist friend, later filled me in on the origin of Premarin. He told me that it is extracted from the urine of pregnant mares. Hence, the name, *pre*gnant plus *mare*! The suffix *in* indicates that it is a medicine.

61. DES continued to be available for veterinary use. It is now formulated by another laboratory, not by Lilly. A chemist friend tells me that he was working at Lilly while DES was being developed. His male colleague, who was working with the formula, absorbed it through his skin and developed oversized breasts. In 2002 we are going through much public scrutiny of hormone replacement therapy for women. The warning labels for Premarin and other such products have always cautioned about possibilities of heart problems and phlebitis. Dr. Logan put it to me this way: "I would rather deal with the slight chance that you might develop some heart problem than with the certainty of advancing prostate cancer."

62. Psalm 22:14-15

63. Gian-Carlo Menotti, *The Medium*, opera in one act.

64. Rachel Naomi Remen, MD, *Kitchen Table Wisdom: Stories That Heal* (New York: Riverhead Books, 1996).

65. Psalm 22:19-21

66. Psalm 22:21b-22

67. Rachel Remen, *Kitchen Table Wisdom*, 80.

68. Meredith Wilson, *The Music Man*, act 2, scene 3 (New York: Music Theater International, 1950, Warner Bros., 1962).

69. Samuel F. Pugh, 1952. Used by permission of the author.

70. American Cancer Society, *Cancer Facts and Figures 2002*, 15.

71. W. J. Catalona, D. S. Smith, and D. K. Ornstein, "Prostate cancer detection in men with serum PSA concentrations of 2.6 to 4.0 ng/ml, and benign prostate examination." *JAMA*, 227:1452-5, 1997. Quoted in *PCR Highlights*, July 2002, vol. 5, no. 1. "First time PSA values of greater than 2.0 are associated with a diagnosis of PC in approximately 20–25 percent of men so studied."

72. Patrick C. Walsh, MD, and Janet Farrar Worthington, *Dr. Patrick Walsh's Guide to Surviving Prostate Cancer* (New York: Warner Books, 2001), 131.

73. It's not as big a deal as you might think. After all, women submit themselves to annual mammograms (my wife calls it "boob-smushing") and vaginal exams. Just give the doc a wide-cheeked smile and relax. It's over in five seconds. I've timed it. It just feels like five minutes.

74. Crittenton Hospital Medical Center Web site, June 8, 2001.

75. Antiangiogenesis: anti=against; angio=vessel; genesis=creation. So antiangiogenesis agents prevent the creation of new blood vessels.

76. As of 2002.

77. The bibliography for this book does not exhaust the resources, but it is fairly current as of this publication date. Resources that are especially useful for factual information are noted with an asterisk (*).